Is Your Voice Telling on You?

How to Find and Use Your Natural Voice

Is Your Voice Telling on You?

How to Find and Use Your Natural Voice

Daniel R. Boone, Ph.D.
Professor Emeritus
Department of Speech and Hearing Sciences
University of Arizona, Tucson, Arizona

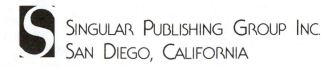
SINGULAR PUBLISHING GROUP INC.
SAN DIEGO, CALIFORNIA

Singular Publishing Group, Inc.
4284 41st Street
San Diego, California 92105

ISBN: 1-879105-03-9

Printed in the United States of America

Contents

Acknowledgments

My thanks to the patients who taught me what to do with voice problems. And to past students in my classes at the University of Arizona. And to the many voice professionals whom I have worked with and learned from over the years. My special thanks to my editor, Bruce Dexter of La Jolla, California, who worked so long and so patiently with me on this book.

Daniel R. Boone, Ph.D.

Preface

When we first hear ourselves on audio- or videotape, a lot of us are embarrassed by the way we sound. "Is that really me?" we ask. In fact, many of us find in both work and social situations that people react to us as if we *were* someone else. Are we creating the impression that we think we are or that we want to?

Sometimes we are aware that our voice is the problem; often we are not. All we know is that people respond to us in ways that frequently surprise and disappoint us, and we pay the price in our careers and personal relationships.

Even when we realize we have some kind of voice problem, most of us do not know precisely what the problem is or what to do about it. We tend to assume that our voice is something we were born with and that we cannot do anything about it.

Is Your Voice Telling on You? will show you that that is not true. It is designed to help those millions of you with poor or ineffective voices to develop better sounding voices. For most of you that will prove to be your *natural voice,* a voice that is distinctively your own, one that makes you sound the way you should.

As a speech pathologist for thirty-five years, I have worked with people with voice problems in hospitals, university clinics, and private practice. Many years ago I began to realize that most poor voices are simply the result of people misusing their natural voice mechanisms. I further observed that most of us sound best when we find our *natural voice,* a voice that allows our physical equipment — our lungs, vocal cords, and resonators — to function as they were designed to function, so that we speak with the right amount of effort, the right breathing, pitch, and balance of relaxation and tension.

Some poor voices are the result of physical disabilities and disease. We call these voice *disorders,* and they are not dealt with in this book. The vast majority of poor voices stem from things that we do, or fail to do, that prevent our natural voices from being heard.

Through a variety of simple self-tests, this book will help you identi-fy what voice problems you have. It will enable you to discover whether they arise from habitual misuse of your vocal equipment, or only in spe-cific circumstances, such as where there is stress or adverse environ-mental factors. For each voice problem we then offer practical exercises to help you correct the problem and begin to use your *natural voice.*

The only aids you will need are an audiocassette recorder, a watch or clock with a second hand, a good listener whom you can call on now and then to listen to you, and a pitch pipe (or piano or guitar for those of you with some musical ability).

The self-tests and the exercises are easy to use. You should be able to hear some improvement in your voice almost immediately, although making that improvement a permanent part of your speaking voice may take a little longer. A good voice, like a good personal appearance or personality, doesn't come with a cosmetic "quick fix," such as running a comb through your hair, or mustering a smile at will. It requires devel-oping a new awareness of the impression you make on others with your voice, and a willingness to train yourself to improve it. It is not difficult to do.

You will enjoy this book, and you will have fun with the self-tests and practice exercises. Most of all, you will enjoy hearing your voice pre-sent you to others as the person you really are. And you will reap the benefits of speaking with your natural voice in your work and your per-sonal relationships.

Daniel R. Boone, Ph.D.

CHAPTER **1**

Your Voice Is Telling On You

"...a beautiful person until she spoke."

We all know people who never get out of their cars without combing their hair, or checking their tie or makeup. They may spend a small fortune on clothes, hairstyling, cosmetics, and fitness. They may have had a fine education, may take night classes, and have read all the books on how to win friends and influence people. Yet all of their efforts can be undone because they have never given much thought to how their voices sound.

You can be confident and always know what you're talking about, and yet your voice sends a different message to others. You can be very fond of another person, respect, admire, even love them, yet your voice inadequately, or incorrectly, reflects such emotions. You can be pleased, angry, excited, worried, sad, but your voice tells a different story.

Granted, there are times when we don't want such feelings to show, and we will discuss this further on in this book. But most of the time it is as important for your voice to mirror your emotions as for your expression to show how you feel. If you want and need people to know who you really are, then you have to send them accurate signals. Voice is one of the principal ways to do this.

Take Ron, age 41, a successful corporate attorney who decided to run for county commissioner. Although he had experienced some hoarseness since his days as a college cheerleader, his rough voice had served him adequately in his law office and his occasional days in court. But when he got into the tough campaign for the commissioner's seat, he became so hoarse that people complained they could not understand him, and what they did understand they weren't sure they liked. During the last week of the campaign, he lost his voice completely. He also lost the election. Following his defeat, Ron decided to do something about his voice. A subsequent evaluation found no physical cause for his voice problem. Rather, it was caused by not using his voice correctly. He spoke at the bottom of his pitch range on inadequate air. Ron began a voice therapy program directed at developing better breathing, a natural pitch, and "an easy voice." After 13 sessions, he could use his newly discovered natural voice in all situations.

How we sound is largely the result of speaking the same way, day after day, over a period of years. If you were lucky enough to develop a good-sounding voice, the luck was related to your having normal vocal equipment — lungs, vocal cords, throat, tongue, jaw, teeth, sinuses — plus being able to use this equipment in an easy, natural way.

Some of us are not that lucky. We might be the man who makes people edgy at a director's meeting because his voice is nasal and tense. We might be the person who sounds so effeminate that other men in the locker room joke about him behind his back. We could be the woman who is mistaken on the telephone for her husband, or the husband who sounds like his wife or mother.

What we sound like is what people think we are.

I remember the case of Rebecca, age 37, a financial consultant for a large investment house. Over a five-year period she had built a list of satisfied clients for various kinds of tax shelters. After the market crash of October 1987, her clients, like most investors, became nervous. So did Rebecca. She was sure her advice was sound, and she had a track record to back her up. But she was under great stress trying to reassure her clients, and her voice showed it. A few customers told her bluntly that she didn't sound convincing. She sought my professional help. I gave her specific voice relaxation techniques to practice, such as the "telephone relaxer" and the "yawn-sigh." I listened to her make a number of calls, and I offered further suggestions for getting back her natural voice on the telephone. By self-practice she reduced her stress-related voice symptoms, and now, again, has what she calls "my old convince-anyone voice."

What both Ron and Rebecca's cases illustrate is that listeners may react more to how you sound than to what you say. The point we made a moment ago is worth repeating: What we sound like is what people think we are.

Your Voice "Fingerprint"

Just like a fingerprint, the human voice and speech pattern is amazingly distinctive. Actually, a few words on the telephone spoken by someone you know, or hearing a friend or family member talking in another room, is all we need to identify who they are.

Our voice "fingerprints" are composed of a number of speech-voice behaviors that act in combination as well as separately.

The Number of Words You Say on One Breath. Some of us say few words on one breath. Some say many. The relative amount of pausing and phrasing that you use becomes unique to you.

How Fast You Speak. The normal conversational speaking rate is about 150 words per minute. If you speak at a different rate, this shapes your individual sound.

Your Rhythm of Speech. Both the number of words you say per breath and your speed of talking contribute to your speech rhythm (or prosody). The melody and speech accents you use in talking, your voice inflections, are distinctively your own.

Your Ease in Breathing. Some of us struggle to have enough breath when we speak. Others never seem to run out of air. Such habitual breathing patterns help give you your vocal identity.

The Pitch of Your Voice. Pitch varies from person to person, even among people of the same age and sex. How high or low your voice is pitched is a major factor in distinguishing your voice from other voices.

The Loudness of Your Voice. Loudness, of course, varies according to the situation in which you speak, but some people normally speak louder, or softer, than others. Your loudness level is also part of your vocal identity.

The Relative Relaxation or Tension of Your Voice. How relaxed or tense you are shows in your voice. The way we sound reflects not only any special circumstances we are in, but also our normal psychological state.

Your Mood State. Vocal individuality also is influenced by such things as whether we are happy or sad, eager, bored, worried, or optimistic.

The Clarity of Your Speech Articulation. Distinctness of speech, or articulation, varies widely from person to person. Some people have distinct accents or dialects. Some have small or large articulation problems, such as not being able to say the *r* sound correctly, or they may have a lisp. Differences of articulation are one of the most noticeable behaviors that distinguish our speech from that of others.

The Resonance of Your Voice. The sound of the voice is heavily influenced by vocal resonance. The position of your tongue, your mouth opening, and the shutting off of your mouth from your nose continually change as you speak and add to your individual sound.

All of these speech-voice behaviors blend together, and what comes out is distinctively you, your individual voice. That is why you can say three words on the telephone and be recognized immediately.

But are you happy with that voice? Ask yourself these three critical questions:

- Are you pleased with your own voice?
- When you hear yourself on a tape recording, do you like the way you sound?
- Generally, do you think your voice makes a good impression on other people?

If the answer to any of these questions is no, then by following a few suggestions in this book and by developing your natural voice through practice, you can become happier with the way you sound and sound better to others.

THE LISTEN TO VOICES TEST

The first step for improving your voice is to develop an awareness of different voices and how they compare with your own. That is the purpose of our Listen to Voices Test.

This six-step test is designed to make you more aware of different voice characteristics. The test begins with an alphabetical list of 100 adjectives, or descriptors, of different voices (see Table 1-1). Each word denotes a positive or negative opinion of a voice. For example, *clear* describes a normal voice free of any kind of defect and is a positive (+) descriptor. The word *scratchy* is a negative (−) descriptor. Some of these terms you will already have heard used to describe voices. Many are seldom used by any of us. And others have their own private meanings for different people.

1. Review the list of 100 word-descriptors. Take time to think about the meaning of each word. Then look at each word and judge it as positive (+) or negative (−), and mark it in the space before each word. Mark even those you are not too sure about. Even if you have never really thought much about voices before, this exercise will help you to develop a better awareness of voice characteristics.

TABLE 1-1. 100 Word-Descriptors for Voice

____ 1. abrasive		____ 35. flat		____ 68. pingy
____ 2. affected		____ 36. feminine		____ 69. pleasing
____ 3. baby		____ 37. fluttering		____ 70. poor
____ 4. bad		____ 38. forced		____ 71. powerful
____ 5. beautiful		____ 39. glassy		____ 72. quivering
____ 6. bell-like		____ 40. golden		____ 73. relaxed
____ 7. blanched		____ 41. good		____ 74. resonant
____ 8. bleaty		____ 42. gravelly		____ 75. rich
____ 9. breathy		____ 43. harmonious		____ 76. ringing
____ 10. bright		____ 44. harsh		____ 77. rough
____ 11. brilliant		____ 45. heady		____ 78. round
____ 12. bubbly		____ 46. heavy		____ 79. scratchy
____ 13. burnished		____ 47. high		____ 80. sexy
____ 14. buzzy		____ 48. hoarse		____ 81. shallow
____ 15. cello-like		____ 49. hollow		____ 82. sharp
____ 16. chesty		____ 50. husky		____ 83. silken
____ 17. clangy		____ 51. immature		____ 84. silvery
____ 18. clear		____ 52. insecure		____ 85. smooth
____ 19. coarse		____ 53. intimidating		____ 86. sophisticated
____ 20. confident		____ 54. light		____ 87. stentorian
____ 21. constricted		____ 55. lovely		____ 88. strident
____ 22. cool		____ 56. low		____ 89. sultry
____ 23. covered		____ 57. macho		____ 90. thin
____ 24. crude		____ 58. masculine		____ 91. throaty
____ 25. cutting		____ 59. mature		____ 92. tight
____ 26. dark		____ 60. mellow		____ 93. timid
____ 27. deep		____ 61. melodious		____ 94. velvety
____ 28. dead		____ 62. metallic		____ 95. warm
____ 29. dry		____ 63. monotone		____ 96. wavering
____ 30. dull		____ 64. nasal		____ 97. wet
____ 31. effeminate		____ 65. open		____ 98. whining
____ 32. effervescent		____ 66. painted		____ 99. whiskey
____ 33. edgy		____ 67. pinched		____ 100. white
____ 34. fearful				

2. Now turn to page 8 at the end of this chapter, and compare your plus or minus markings with mine. There are no right or wrong answers, but the list was designed to include 50 positive modifiers and 50 negative ones. Some words, like *burnished* or *glassy* or *effervescent*, force you to search inside yourself for what such a voice would sound like.

3. Now, see if you can apply some of these voice-descriptors to the voices of famous people you have heard in the movies or on television. Selecting the words that might apply to a well-known voice can help you learn to listen more critically to the voices around you. Go through the list below and apply the words that you think describe the voice of each celebrity. I have listed my choices of descriptive words for each. Do you agree or disagree with me?

Tom Brokaw:	bright, confident, good, low, masculine, melodious, resonant, throaty
George Burns:	bad, burnished, gravelly, hoarse, husky, rough, scratchy, whiskey
George Bush:	clangy, confident, metallic, nasal, pingy, ringing, strident
William Buckley:	burnished, cello-like, cool, deep, golden, heavy, melodious, relaxed, resonant, sophisticated, velvety
Walter Cronkite:	brilliant, clear, confident, open, ringing, strident, warm
Goldie Hawn:	baby, bubbly, feminine, immature, light, pleasing, sexy, wavering
James Earl Jones:	bell-like, clear, deep, golden, low, melodious, powerful, resonant
Marilyn Monroe:	affected, breathy, feminine, relaxed, sexy, sultry, wet
Meryl Streep:	bright, clear, cool, good, pleasing, sharp, warm
Barbara Walters:	abrasive, affected, burnished, clangy, friendly, intimidating (at times), sophisticated, whining

My descriptors for the voices of these well-known people may differ from yours. That is all right. The important part of this exercise is to apply descriptive labels to help you become more aware of the different-sounding voices around you.

Now, what about your own voice?

4. Listen to your own voice. Tape record your reading or improvising a paragraph or two. As you listen to the playback, select from the list of 100 descriptors seven or eight of the words that you think best describe your voice. Then listen to the playback again, and narrow your list down to three descriptors. These three words describe your voice as you hear it.

5. Ask a close friend, or your spouse, to review the 100-word list, and then to select the seven or eight words he or she thinks best describe your voice. Were your final three descriptors among those selected by this other person?

6. Select five or six other voices that you have heard, either in person or on radio or television. If you can, tape record these voices and listen to the playback critically. Once again, review the 100-word list and select the word that best describes each voice.

By completing the six steps above, you will start to become aware of the individuality of the voices around you. You will develop a better awareness of your own voice. And you will develop a better awareness of which qualities of voices are pleasing to hear and which are not.

How to Find Your Natural Voice

Unfortunately, although many people realize that their voices don't represent them well, either generally or in special circumstances, they don't know what to do to change the way they sound or how to find their natural voices.

Each of us *has* a natural voice. It is a voice that uses our physical vocal equipment in an easy, efficient manner, that achieves a natural balance of breathing, phonation (the way the vocal cords vibrate), and resonance.

In the following chapters we will show you the various ways to find the natural voice that is distinctively your own. We will show you how to develop and maintain it and tell you what to do to avoid a bad voice, even in stressful situations.

But first we need to understand the voice mechanisms that control the way we sound.

TABLE 1-2. Author's Ratings of 100 Word-Descriptors for Voice

—	1. abrasive	—	35. flat	—	68. pingy
—	2. affected	+	36. feminine	+	69. pleasing
—	3. baby	—	37. fluttering	—	70. poor
—	4. bad	—	38. forced	+	71. powerful
+	5. beautiful	+	39. glassy	—	72. quivering
+	6. bell-like	+	40. golden	+	73. relaxed
+	7. blanched	+	41. good	+	74. resonant
—	8. bleaty	—	42. gravelly	+	75. rich
+	9. breathy	+	43. harmonious	+	76. ringing
+	10. bright	—	44. harsh	—	77. rough
+	11. brilliant	—	45. heady	+	78. round
+	12. bubbly	—	46. heavy	—	79. scratchy
+	13. burnished	+	47. high	+	80. sexy
—	14. buzzy	—	48. hoarse	—	81. shallow
+	15. cello-like	—	49. hollow	—	82. sharp
+	16. chesty	—	50. husky	+	83. silken
—	17. clangy	—	51. immature	+	84. silvery
+	18. clear	—	52. insecure	+	85. smooth
—	19. coarse	—	53. intimidating	+	86. sophisticated
+	20. confident	+	54. light	+	87. stentorian
—	21. constricted	+	55. lovely	—	88. strident
+	22. cool	+	56. low	+	89. sultry
+	23. covered	+	57. macho	—	90. thin
—	24. crude	+	58. masculine	—	91. throaty
—	25. cutting	+	59. mature	—	92. tight
—	26. dark	+	60. mellow	—	93. timid
+	27. deep	+	61. melodious	+	94. velvety
—	28. dead	—	62. metallic	+	95. warm
—	29. dry	—	63. monotone	—	96. wavering
—	30. dull	—	64. nasal	+	97. wet
—	31. effeminate	+	65. open	—	98. whining
+	32. effervescent	+	66. painted	—	99. whiskey
—	33. edgy	—	67. pinched	+	100. white
—	34. fearful				

CHAPTER **2**

The Basic Mechanisms of the Natural Voice

"I could listen to him all day long."

For a lifetime most of us use the same voice, regardless of the situations in which we find ourselves, regardless of whether it pleases us or others, and regardless of whether it gives an accurate impression of who we really are. We take our voices for granted, as something given, like the shape of our nose or the size of our feet. As one patient said to me, "I've had this lousy voice all my life, and no one ever told me I could fix it." But the voice can be changed just as our appearance, intellect, and personality can.

There is no magic required. Developing a voice that sounds better entails learning to use one's breathing mechanisms, vocal cords, and resonating cavities in a natural manner. We call this voice produced with very little effort your natural voice. For most of us, it is there waiting to be used.

The natural voice requires a natural balance between the basic mechanisms of breathing, phonation (vocal cord vibration), and resonance. Before we look more closely at each mechanism, let us look at three people who lacked such a natural balance: Billy Joe, who was too concerned about his breathing; Agnes, who put too much effort into phonation; and Jamie, who had too much throat resonance. The careers of each of these people suffered because of the way they sounded. Each received voice therapy and found his or her natural voice.

Billy Joe was a 28-year-old aspiring disc jockey who unnecessarily lost his first job because of a poor voice. While broadcasting, he became overly conscious of taking in air. He elevated his shoulders, lifted his chin, pushed out his stomach, and made audible sounds while inhaling. His breathing problem came directly from all the unnecessary things that he did to "assist" his breathing. The result was audible voice strain. His station manager had to let him go after listeners complained that "he sounded as if he'd run five miles to get to the microphone." It took six months of voice therapy to restore his natural ability to breathe while speaking, breathing that required no monitoring or special effort. All Billy Joe had to do was learn to pause now and then. When he paused, the breath cycle renewed itself with no special effort on his part. When he learned to do this, Billy Joe was on his way to another radio station.

Agnes was a 61-year-old realtor whose voice had taken an elevator ride to the bottom of her range. Her voice became so low-pitched that her realty clients began to have difficulty understanding her. When she came to our voice clinic, we soon discovered that she could not speak at a lower pitch even if she wanted to. Agnes told us that she felt her voice pitch had lowered after her menopause (a common occurrence that is described in Chapter 13). She also felt her condition was related to the fact that she had been a heavy smoker much of her adult life, although she no longer smoked. In short, in Agnes' mind, the changes in her voice were inevitable because of her age and smoking.

They weren't. To improve her voice, we recommended two things. First, she should speak about three notes higher. It turned out that she could do this with a little practice. Second, she needed to lift the focus of her voice out of her throat and into her mouth. This second therapy goal used imagery. We asked her to "think of your mouth as a big cathedral. We want your voice sounding up in the ceiling." Such imagery, which is more fully described in Chapter 8, immediately helped her produce a more natural voice. When she learned to speak at the higher pitch levels, and with greater vertical focus, her hoarseness disappeared, and she was easier to understand.

Then there was *Jamie,* a 26-year-old salesman, who had had a bad voice all of his life. Recently, he had become aware that his voice was hurting him in his sales work. It came from so far back in his throat that as a boy he was teased for sounding like Mortimer Snerd. On voice examination, we found that Jamie's problem was throat resonance, caused by his tongue being excessively retracted in his mouth. His adult voice sounded somewhat like the television character Alf (not much of an improvement over Mortimer Snerd). Some of his front-of-the-mouth speech sounds, such as *th* and *t*, were slightly compromised by his back-in-the-mouth focus. In voice therapy, he did exercises designed to bring his tongue forward (as described in Chapter 8). Jamie practiced these tongue movements throughout the day. As his tongue was carried more toward the middle of his mouth, his voice resonance improved dramatically, and Jamie at last discovered his natural voice.

Almost anyone with normal vocal equipment (as was true of Billy Joe, Agnes, and Jamie) can achieve a natural voice with very little effort — in fact, trying to use a voice that isn't really your own strains your vocal equipment.

A natural voice is produced with easy breathing, at a pitch level that takes little muscular effort in the larynx, and resonates nicely in an open throat and mouth. The three components of voice — breathing, phonation, and resonance — work in a balanced, almost effortless way.

Before we examine each component in detail, we need to speak for a moment about controlling your voice on those occasions when control is important. Your natural voice generally reflects the way you really feel. If you are happy, you sound happy. If you are angry, your listeners hear it in your voice. In most situations our voices *should* reveal how we feel. But certainly not in all situations. For example, an airline captain facing a difficult landing cannot let passengers hear the fear in his voice. Or the executive who feels great tension when making an important presentation does not want his or her voice to betray anxiety.

There are times, then, when we must control our natural voice so that it represents us the way we want to appear, rather than the way we feel. Parents do this a lot of the time with their children. It is called voice control. In addition to developing a natural voice (the basic message of this book), we will also learn ways to control the natural voice in special situations, such as on the telephone or when suffering from stage fright or stress.

But, back to the three mechanisms of voice: breathing, phonation, and resonance. How does each contribute to the natural voice?

Breathing and the Natural Voice

All speech is produced on expiratory air. When we speak, we take in a quick, momentary breath and then let it out slowly. The air makes our vocal cords vibrate (phonation). But the body's need for oxygen renewal will always take precedence over our attempts to talk. For example, as we climb a mountain trail, we will speak in short gasps, despite our efforts to speak in one long, smooth sentence. Or, if we are involved in a tense situation, such as an auto accident, the brain will signal for more oxygen in the emergency, and our normal speech will suffer — sometimes to the point that when someone asks us, "What happened?" we literally cannot tell them.

Breathing for speech differs from the regular in-and-out breathing we use when reading silently or sleeping. That quick breath that we take to speak comes from a sudden expansion of the chest, and the lungs within it, by using chest muscles and the downward descent of the diaphragm (see Figure 2-1). As the chest muscles relax, and the diaphragm relaxes, the chest and lungs get smaller. This decrease in the size of both lungs increases the air pressure within them, and the air is exhaled.

FIGURE 2-1. Breathing Mechanisms. Air from the nose and mouth passes through the larynx (1), through the windpipe or trachea (2), and on into the lungs (3). The air is distributed through the lungs via the bronchial tubes (4). The large diaphragm (5), which separates the chest from the abdomen, is the primary muscle of inspiration.

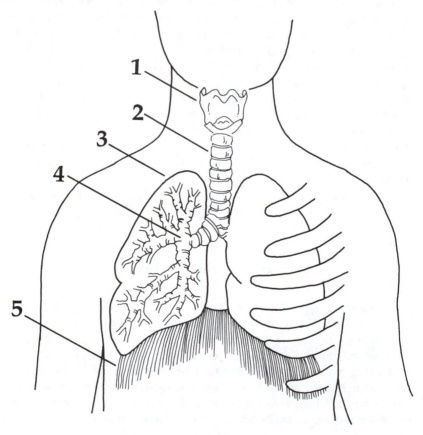

When we start to run out of air as we are speaking, we need to pause, as we saw in the case of Billy Joe. During the pause our chest expands again, we take in a new breath, and we are able to continue talking. The muscle movements required in the breath cycle take care of themselves automatically during the pause.

The loudness of your voice is controlled by your breathing too. A whisper requires very little outgoing air. The louder the voice, the more air we use.

The key to breathing for producing a natural voice is to do it effortlessly. Most of us need no special training in breathing. Contrary to what many people think, we do not have to learn diaphragmatic breathing to develop a good voice. All we need to do is become aware of how many words we can say with average loudness on one breath. Then, as we are talking, we need to *pause* before we get to this upper limit of words per breath, and the body will renew the breath it needs.

Phonation and the Natural Voice

The outgoing airstream passes out of the lungs, via the bronchial tubes and the trachea, into the larynx. (These structures can be seen in Figure 2-1.) The two vocal cords are in the larynx. As we see in Figure 2-2, the vocal cords are usually in one of two positions.

In sketch A, we see the two vocal cords apart, like an inverted V. This is the position they are in during breathing; the air passes between them without obstruction. For phonation, they come together as seen in sketch B. In this closed position, the outgoing airstream passes between the vocal cords and starts them vibrating. As they vibrate, the vocal cords

FIGURE 2-2. The vocal cords. A. The two vocal cords are open in an inverted V. B. The vocal cords are together for voicing (phonation).

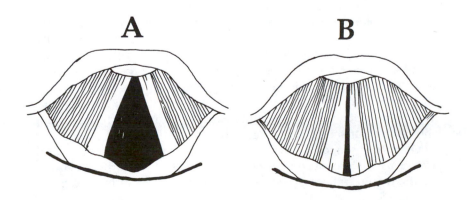

A   B

make a noise that voice scientists and speech pathologists call phonation. We know it better as voice.

The natural voice can be produced only when the vocal cords are gently together. If they are too far apart, the voice is likely to be breathy. Vocal cords that are held together too tightly result in a harsh voice. A gentle proximity of the vocal cords produces the desired easy voice. You probably already produce it now and then. For example, when you say "uhm huh," this gentle sound of agreement is probably your natural voice, easy and relaxed.

The pitch of your voice is determined by the thickness, size, and tension of your vocal cords. Large, relaxed vocal cords produce low pitches. Thin, tense vocal cords produce high pitches. We cannot voluntarily change the shape of our vocal cords. We don't need to. As we speak, and certainly as we sing, the vocal cords constantly change size. The muscles in the larynx and the vocal cords, which are a pair of muscles themselves, contract or relax automatically to produce the pitch we want to use.

The natural pitch of the voice, that easy "uhm huh" sound, can be produced with very little effort. It seems to exist several notes above the bottom of our total range. This natural pitch level is an important part of our natural voice, and we will talk about it in detail in Chapter 7.

Resonance and the Natural Voice

The resonance of the voice is produced primarily in the cavities above the vocal cords: the throat, mouth, and nose. The primary resonance cavity is the pharynx, or throat. The lateral and posterior walls of the throat are sphincteric muscles. When they contract, the pharynx becomes smaller (as it does in singing a high note). When these constrictor muscles relax, the pharynx becomes larger (as in using a low voice). A natural voice seems to require an open, relaxed throat.

Much voice resonance also occurs in the mouth. Accordingly, the position of the tongue in the mouth has a great deal of influence on how we sound. A tongue that is carried far forward in the mouth can produce a baby-like voice. A backward carriage of the tongue produces a back focus to the voice, like Jamie the salesman's, altering one's resonance to sound almost like the television character Alf. A vocal coach in New York City told me that a voice with good resonance sounds as if "it's coming right off the surface of the tongue in the middle of the mouth."

Only three sounds in English, *m, n, ng*, require nasal resonance. Nasal resonance is produced by sound waves traveling into the nasal cavities. The mouth and nasal cavities are separated by the bony hard palate (the front roof of the mouth) and the muscular soft palate (the back roof of the mouth). In normal speech, without *m, n,* or *ng,* the soft palate door to the nasal cavities remains closed. When we say the nasal sounds, this door quickly opens, by dropping down. The sound waves then have to travel through the soft palate door into the nasal cavities. As we will discuss in Chapter 9, some of us have too much nasal resonance, and some of us have too little. The natural voice has the right balance between oral and nasal resonance.

How to Tell if You Have a Voice Problem

A *voice disorder* is not the same as a voice problem. By a voice disorder we mean something that needs to be treated by a specialist. A conservative estimate of the percentage of voice disorders in adults (there has never been a national survey) is that about three percent of the population in this country over age 18 has a voice disorder of some kind. Some of the specialists listed in Chapter 16 are the best qualified professionals to help these seven million Americans with voice disorders.

But probably 25 percent of the adult population, although they do not have real voice disorders, are displeased with the way they sound and with the way their voices affect their careers and social lives. Their problems undoubtedly are with one or more of the elements of a natural voice that we have been discussing. Based on the 1986 census figures, that means well over 60 million Americans may have voice problems.

Are you one of them? Take a few moments now to take the Voice Self-Analysis Test that follows. It will give you some insight into how real your concern about the way you sound is.

VOICE SELF-ANALYSIS TEST

This test contains 20 statements. Read and consider each one. Then mark each statement true (+) or false (−), according to your view of your voice.

_____ 1. You frequently find that you are short of breath as you speak.

_____ 2. You don't like to listen to yourself on a tape recording.

_____ 3. Your voice gets tired as you use it.

_____ 4. Strangers on the telephone think you are younger or older than you are.

_____ 6. Your voice is different in the morning than it is at night.

_____ 7. After you talk a lot, your throat hurts.

_____ 8. People have difficulty hearing you in some situations.

_____ 9. Your voice doesn't sound as good as it used to sound.

_____ 10. Your voice sounds as if it is in your nose.

_____ 11. Your voice sounds as if you are nervous.

_____ 12. You may lose your voice when you are nervous or tired.

_____ 13. When you speak, you don't have the voice you want.

_____ 14. You would like to change the pitch of your voice.

_____ 15. You feel that your voice isn't "really you."

_____ 16. You frequently clear your throat.

_____ 17. When you have an allergy or a cold, you sometimes lose your voice.

_____ 18. Your throat feels excessively dry and scratchy after prolonged speaking.

_____ 19. People frequently misunderstand what you say.

_____ 20. Strangers on the telephone think you are of the opposite sex.

Check the 20 statements again to see if your first answers truly represent how you feel about your voice. Now, count up the number of true answers. Most of us will have a concern or two (a few true answers) about our voices.

After administering this test to a number of adults, I was able to rate the degree of concern about voice on the following scale:

Number of True Answers	Amount of Concern
0–2	No concern
3–4	Mild concern
5–8	Moderate concern
9 or more	Severe concern

The higher your degree of concern, the more probable it is that you are using a voice that is different from your natural voice.

If you are concerned about your voice, do something about it. In the following chapters you will find out what environmental and physical factors can adversely affect your voice and what you, yourself, may be doing to adversely affect it. Once these problems are identified, you will learn what to do about them. As you will see, learning to use an easy voice, free of effort, is not that difficult.

CHAPTER 3

Enemies of a Natural Voice

"The problem may not be your fault,
but not doing anything about it is."

In this chapter we will look at possible environmental and physical enemies to having a better voice. You may not be able to eliminate them entirely, but when you encounter them, you need to know how to cope with them to minimize their negative impact on your voice.

Environmental Enemies of a Natural Voice

There are five principal environmental enemies of a natural voice:

Air quality	dust, fumes, smoke, smog
Special circumstances	telephones, microphones, cars, planes, public speaking
Humidity	low or high moisture levels in the air you breathe
Noise	recreational, occupational, travel, and extraneous noise
Speaker-listener distance	too close, too far, large room, and outside speaking

Air Quality Problems. The most common air quality problem is not smog, but dust. Dust from chalk, from the carpet, household dust, backstage dust, outside dust blown into your home or office from passing cars, construction projects, leaf blowers.

Dust is an irritant to your airway, the wet or moist linings of your nose, throat, and vocal cords. When irritated, these air passages may become red and swollen, often causing a change in the pitch and quality of your voice.

Indoor dusting can do wonders to reduce this problem. I remember an actress telling me, "After they started wet-mopping the stage and backstage floors before the show, my voice problems disappeared."

Do what you can to reduce the dust in your home, office, or other work places. Although you cannot eliminate outside dust from sources beyond your control, it can be reduced around your home by plantings and by watering down dusty areas. In some foreign countries, such as Spain and Italy, during the dry, dusty months of summer, you can see shopkeepers and homeowners sprinkling water on the sidewalks in front of their shops and homes to keep down the dust.

The smog in our cities from the emissions of cars, trucks, buses, and industry and the smoke from fireplaces and barbecues are definite irritants to your airway.

Inside the house or work place, air conditioning can make a big difference. Air conditioning units in cars are perhaps more important for their air filtering properties than for their cooling. I knew a drugstore salesman in Los Angeles who cured his chronic hoarseness by adding an air conditioning unit to his car.

Become more aware of air quality as a potential enemy of your voice. If bad air is present, drink more fluids, stay indoors more, and see if you can add air conditioning to your living and work spaces.

Special Circumstances. There are certain common situations that seem to work against having a natural voice, and they vary from individual to individual. Some people have difficulty using their natural voice on the telephone. They clear their throats often, become short of breath, and even use a different voice. This is a much more common problem than you might think; many people dislike talking on the telephone at all. Because so many people have a voice problem using the telephone, we have included a separate chapter (Chapter 12) on this topic. In that chapter, we also talk about how to keep your natural voice when using a microphone.

Some people find that talking before groups, or speaking with a supervisor, can have a negative effect on their voices. Chapters 10 through 14 contain tips for situations like these.

Automobiles and airplanes are common places where people have voice problems, not only because such environments are noisy but because they can be excessively dry. On long car trips, we should avoid protracted conversations and carry a supply of soft drinks or water. Airplane cabins are also often too dry, and good fluid intake during air travel helps prevent not only jet lag, but voice problems as well. These concerns are of particular importance to people who are expected to speak at the end of a long journey, perhaps at a conference or meeting, in a lecture, or during a sales call.

Humidity. Too low or too high humidity can be an enemy of your natural voice. An ideal humidity for the voice is between 40 and 50 percent. In desert areas, such as Tucson or Palm Springs, humidity levels frequently drop below 10 percent. This dries out the air passages in the vocal tract. The mucosal surfaces of the mouth and throat become excessively dry, often showing red streaks or inflammation. In such circumstances, we need to drink far more fluids and add moisture to the air. Inside, humidity can be raised by swamp coolers, humidifiers, or by keeping well-watered house plants around.

Humidity levels above 85 percent may add too much moisture to our airways, which can cause us to continually clear our throats and blow our noses. In cars, homes, and offices, excessive humidity can be controlled somewhat by using air conditioners and furnaces that have dehumidifiers. Unfortunately, many of these units remove too much moisture from the air. Remember, humidity levels around 40 to 50 percent seem to be best for the voice. Most hardware stores sell gauges that show humidity as well as temperature levels.

Noise. Some people call this the biggest air pollutant of all. And often, the sources of smog and dust — cars, construction projects, blowers — are also sources of noise pollution.

In everyday life, we frequently find ourselves in noisy places, in cars, planes, trains, buses, subways, restaurants, discos, stadiums, around power mowers and blowers, construction sites, or just on the sidewalks of a busy city street. We need to be careful about prolonged speaking in such circumstances. When we speak in a noisy situation, generally we are unaware of how loudly we are talking. Many of us have had the experience of having music, or conversation, stop suddenly when we are talking. We are surprised to find we are almost shouting.

The extra effort required to speak in noisy environments involves using more air for a louder voice, a higher pitch, and greater precision in enunciation. This can severely tax our vocal equipment and prevent us from using our natural voices.

One noisy situation worth special mention is wearing a Walkman headset. Avoid using your voice much when listening to your Walkman. The noise level is usually too high for you to speak at your normal level.

Speaker-Listener Distance. Most of us use many different voices every day, depending on how near or far we are from our listeners. At close distances, we speak at a low loudness level. When we stand before a group, our listeners are farther away, and we need to take a bigger breath to speak loudly and to use fewer words per breath.

For a good voice, and one that can be heard effectively, we need to vary our loudness to meet the situation and not use the same loudness level wherever we are. In Chapter 6, Loud Enough or Too Loud?, we will look at ways to find the loudness levels appropriate for various speaker-listener distances.

Physical Enemies of a Natural Voice

In addition to environmental threats to the natural voice, there are some physical factors that influence how we sound. The eight conditions listed below may be major enemies of developing and using your natural voice.

Aging	The voice changes throughout our lifespan.
Allergies and infections	Common ailments change our voices.
Fatigue	Tiredness quickly shows in our voices.
Fear	Being afraid affects our airway.
Hormonal changes	Glandular changes influence the voice.
Hydration	Moisture levels in the airway and the vocal tract affect the voice.
Medications	Some medicines may impact on the voice.
Recreational drugs	Smoking, alcohol, and illegal drugs have an impact on our voices.

Aging. Voice mirrors physical growth and other changes of the body. At age 9, boys and girls basically have the same voice pitch, near middle C on a musical scale. With the advent of puberty, the male voice drops an octave, and the female voice half an octave. A man's voice continues to deepen as he gets older, until past age 70 when his voice pitch begins to elevate slightly. The adult female voice tends to get lower in pitch with each successive decade. In very old age, past age 90, the voice pitches of men and women are relatively similar.

As we get older, our rate of speech also generally slows a bit from the 150 words a minute of our younger days. An older man once asked me, "How can I sound younger?" I told him, "Listen to Bob Hope. Here is a man in his mid-eighties who uses a slightly higher pitch, and speaks rapidly, and this makes his speech patterns sound young."

Allergies and Infections. The professional user of voice (and this includes not just actors, singers, preachers, and teachers, but all of us who need to use our voices effectively in our daily work) is always fearful of an allergy or infection that might temporarily put his or her voice our of commission.

For people with severe airway allergies, the swollen and inflamed membranes of the throat and nose can produce hoarseness and even complete loss of voice. The best source of treatment for allergies is a physician, either an allergist or an ear-nose-throat specialist. Be wary of taking over-the-counter allergy medications, such as antihistamines, on your own. Most antihistamines have profound drying effects on the larynx, which may only add to the deterioration of voice.

Most throat infections are viral in origin, and are difficult to treat. The best thing we can do when a severe cold affects our voice is to rest and take extra fluids, particularly citrus juices. If we sound hoarse, we should go on complete voice rest for a few days, using no voice at all. Talking a lot with a voice hoarse from a cold can damage the vocal cords. Voice rest will allow the infected cords to heal. (If a severe head cold lingers more than seven days, you should see a doctor.)

Fatigue. We all know the symptoms of physical fatigue: we want to lie down, perhaps have a drink of some kind, and most of us want to be left alone. If we are forced to speak to someone, our voice is light, higher in pitch, and lower in volume than usual. At these times, it is not always possible to have the kind of voice you would like to have. Yet with rest, and a proper diet, it is amazing how quickly your voice will come back. If you need to use your voice when fatigued, elevate your pitch a note and speak a bit faster. Adding a higher focus to your voice (see Chapter 8) can also make a fatigued voice sound more alive.

Fear. When we are afraid, the body alerts a number of physical systems to be ready to respond to danger. Our breathing rate increases, our heartbeat accelerates, our blood pressure goes up, the larynx tends to elevate, and the vocal folds often form a tight protective sphincter.

All of the above body postures help the body make a realistic response to a fearful situation. The problem is, however, that most of the time we don't need such forceful reactions, yet the voice gives out the sounds of fear. It sounds tense and has a higher pitch, and we say fewer words than normal per breath. In Chapter 11, Stage Fright and Other Fears, we talk about things we can do to take the sound of fear out of our voices, for example, a big yawn followed by a sigh.

Hormonal Changes. The dramatic voice changes in puberty experienced by both boys and girls, are obvious evidence of the impact of sex hormones on the vocal tract and are normal. The adult male and female pitch levels stay about half an octave apart throughout most of life. However, the adult female may experience some special fluctuations in pitch (see Chapter 13, The Woman and Her Voice) during menstruation and after the menopause as a direct result of normal hormonal changes.

There are some abnormal hormonal barriers to the natural voice. The adrenal glands can become underproductive, which keeps voice pitch at high, prepubertal levels, or overproductive, which markedly lowers voice. Diseases of the pituitary glands can retard laryngeal growth. An inactive thyroid gland can lower pitch, give a low focus to the voice, and reduce normal loudness. Hyperthyroidism can result in rapid speech and elevated voice pitch. Pitch levels that are inappropriate for an individual's age and sex may be the result of some kind of hormonal imbalance. All such abnormal conditions are best treated by an endocrinologist.

Hydration. Careful attention to moisture levels in both inspired air and the body is essential to a normal voice. Most of us need to drink more fluids, water, coffee, juice, tea, or soft drinks. A dry vocal tract will not function as well as a moist one. Fluids increase saliva and moisture in the airway, from your nostrils down to the bronchial tubes in your lungs. Also, the air that we breathe should, as we noted earlier, contain about 40 to 50 percent humidity to prevent vocal tract dryness.

Without adequate hydration, our voices sound strained and lack their normal resonance. The throat will not only feel dry, but there may be pain. With adequate intake of fluids, the sound of the voice can improve, and throat dryness and pain can disappear. For the occasional person who suffers from excessive mouth dryness, there are several over-the-counter preparations that are helpful for increasing mouth saliva. Ask your pharmacist about them.

Medications. Among over-the-counter drugs, the primary enemies of the vocal tract are aspirin and antihistamines. Continuous and heavy use of aspirin can result in slight hemorrhaging of small blood vessels on the vocal cords, which will lower pitch and produce some hoarseness. Antihistamines tend to dry the throat excessively and make prolonged speaking almost impossible.

Most prescription drugs will not hurt your voice. However, among those that can change your voice are the diuretics (frequently used by dieters), which can excessively dry the airway. Also, some drugs used in the treatment of hypertension to lower blood pressure can have drying effects. Some of the Beta-block drugs, which are prescribed for heart problems, have voice-related side effects, such as throat spasms or sudden loss of voice. Prescription hormones can cause difficulty in breath control, pitch, and voice quality.

You need to be aware of the voice-changing side effects of prescription drugs. If you are taking such a drug, ask your physician or pharmacist about it.

Recreational Drugs. Smoking is a primary enemy of developing a better voice. Cigarette, cigar, and pipe smoke have profound drying effects on the vocal tract, and the tars and irritants in the smoke often cause irritation of the mucosal linings of the air passages. Smoking can cause shortness of breath, coughing, throat clearing, lowering of voice pitch, and decrease in voice loudness. After a habitual smoker stops smoking, many of these symptoms fortunately begin to clear up. It should be pointed out that many, but not all, mild-to-moderate smokers never experience any voice difficulties, but they are surely playing the wrong side of the odds.

Mild (one drink daily) to moderate (two to three drinks) use of alcohol does not seem to harm the natural voice. But heavy use (three or more drinks a day) acts as a vasodilator, enlarging the small blood vessels of the vocal cords, and can result in a husky or rough, low-pitched voice, the "whiskey tenor."

Among illegal drugs, marijuana, when smoked often, can have pronounced drying effects on the membranes of the throat and larynx. Cocaine can cause severe vasoconstriction (shrinking) of the membranes of the nose, resulting in changes of vocal resonance, such as increased nasality.

Along with health and legal consequences, the serious user of voice should consider the potentially harmful effects on the voice from smoking, heavy use of alcohol, and use of illegal drugs such as marijuana or cocaine.

CHAPTER 4

You and Your Natural Voice

"We have met the enemy and he is us."

— Walt Kelly

This quote from Walt Kelly's *Pogo* seems to apply to a great deal of human behavior, and voice production is no exception. While the physical and environmental factors we discussed in the last chapter can profoundly affect how well you speak, the biggest enemy of your natural voice is usually your own vocal behavior. Habitual misuse of vocal equipment invariably results in voice strain, and over a period of time, that strain may create voice problems.

The following simple descriptive list of poor vocal behaviors may help you identify the source of your own problems.

What You May Be Doing to Prevent a Natural Voice

Clenched teeth	You speak through clenched teeth.
Hard glottal attack	You use too much effort to speak
Loudness problems	You speak too loudly or too softly.
Nasality	You speak through your nose too much.
Pitch problems	Your voice is pitched too high or too low.
Running out of air	You don't budget your air for speaking.
Talk, talk, talk	You talk so much that your voice gets tired.
Throat focus	You speak too low in your throat.

Posture problems	You sit or stand improperly.
Stressful environments	Under stress you make inappropriate demands on your voice.
Misinformation	Poor information about your voice causes you to create, or persist in, voice problems.

Clenched Teeth. Every now and then you see someone who speaks with his teeth clenched together, using almost no jaw or lip movement, like a ventriloquist.

This clenched-teeth way of talking puts great strain on the vocal tract. It takes a lot of muscular effort to speak with such restricted mouth and jaw movements. Lack of mouth and jaw movement forces the tongue to do all the work. The voice comes out muffled, speech can be indistinct, and listeners can get the impression that the speaker is reluctant to communicate at all.

To counteract this, there are techniques that encourage jaw and lip movement, such as the open-mouth and yawn-sign exercises described in Chapters 10 and 11.

Hard Glottal Attack. The abruptness that we use when speaking is known as *glottal attack.* The glottis is the space between the vocal cords. Glottal attack is the term we use to describe how quickly the vocal cords close the glottal space. A *soft* glottal attack is heard in the mild, easy speech of the true Southerner. Vowels are prolonged, and the overall speech pattern sounds easy and relaxed. The opposite speech pattern is a crisp, forceful (and frequently forced) way of speaking. Voice scientists and speech pathologists label this a *hard* glottal attack.

We hear the hard attack often in the big cities of the northeastern United States, or when we listen to many television interviewers and newscasters. It is a voice that sounds impersonal and, like the loud voice described below, keeps listeners at a distance. The hard glottal attack takes a toll on the voice, often causing vocal strain and hoarseness. Most of the subsequent chapters of this book give you techniques to eliminate such a hard glottal attack.

Loudness Problems. The loudness of our voices should continually adjust to the changing noise levels around us, to the physical distance between us and our listeners, and to the social circumstances we are in. Unfortunately, many of us habitually use the same level of loudness, regardless of where we are, and consistently speak too loudly or too softly. An inappropriately loud voice can affront or intimidate listeners. The more common too-soft voice is often irritatingly indistinct.

You can change your voice loudness primarily by changing the amount of air you take in before you speak and by adjusting the number of words you say on one breath. But there are many other techniques that can be used too. Chapter 6, Loud Enough or Too Loud?, describes exercises that will help a voice that is too soft or too loud.

Nasality. Another major speaking problem is a nasal-sounding voice. Some voices are so nasal that it is difficult to understand what is said. The problem seems aggravated when the speaker uses a public address system, and in places like hospitals and airports, a nasal voice can create real difficulties. Also, nasal voices are simply irritating — and can be yet another reason why people don't listen to *what* you say because of *how* you say it.

In many ways, a nasal voice is a voice with an excessively high focus. The focus is so high that it is in the nose. Because so many of our voices are too nasal, Chapter 9, Talking Through Your Nose, is devoted to techniques for reducing voice nasality.

Pitch Problems. The natural pitch level we use when we answer "uhm huh" to someone we are talking with is usually near our natural pitch level. Many of us, however, customarily use a voice that is pitched higher or lower than that, and such a voice is produced with some strain on the vocal tract.

Pitch is one of the major voice characteristics that establishes your vocal identity and personality. We are identified not only by our overall pitch level, but by the way we vary pitch within conversational passages — our pattern of speech inflections. A voice that is pitched too high or too low on the telephone can cause the person on the other end of the line to think we are someone else, or even to be confused about what sex we are. A voice that doesn't use inflections is a monotonous, tiring voice, while an overinflected voice can be distracting and irritating to listen to.

Sometimes changing your pitch only one note up or down can add attractiveness and a relaxed sound to the way you speak. For those who speak too softly, raising pitch one note can take the strain out of speaking loudly enough to be heard. And varying your pitch for inflected speech can make all the difference in whether people find what you say interesting or dull. The exercises presented in Chapter 7, The Well-Aimed Pitch, such as the "uhm huh," can keep your listeners from responding, "ho hum."

Running Out of Air. Although it happens all the time, it doesn't make sense that a person runs out of breath when speaking. From the moment of birth, our breathing apparatus is totally automatic. Awake or asleep, when we need air, our bodies simply take it in, adjusting for situations when we need more air (exercising) and less air (sleeping). But when it comes to speaking, many of us try to become do-it-yourselfers. That makes about as much sense as crawling under the hood of your car and moving the engine pistons up and down by hand.

Voice is produced by outgoing breath. For speech, we take in a bit more air than we do for normal breathing. Problems arise when that first breath isn't big enough to sustain all the words we want to say. It is at this point that many of us seem to forget that the breathing process is automatic. We go on trying to speak, with a tight, strangled voice, or we start racing to the end of a sentence with our voice getting increasingly faint, when all we ever have to do is pause. For those of you with breathing problems, *pause* is the magic word. When you do, your body automatically takes in more air, your lungs fill again, and you are ready to speak more words in an easy, natural manner.

We talk about breathing for the speaking voice in the next chapter, To Breathe or Not To Breathe, and show you how to find out how many words you can comfortably say on one breath.

Talk, Talk, Talk. Some people never seem to stop talking. They act as if the sound of their voices is the only thing that keeps them visible to those around them. At the least, they seem more interested in what they say than in what anyone else might say — although sometimes we wonder if they even listen to themselves.

On the other hand, many of us are in occupations that require an enormous amount of talking: teachers, sales persons, air traffic controllers, actors, announcers, telephone receptionists. Still more of us have occupations where we periodically need to do a great deal of talking, such as being called on to make presentations, demonstrate products or systems, or speak at meetings or conferences.

For all heavy users of voice, whether occasional or frequent, it is essential to speak in as natural a manner as possible. Poor voice behavior can cause strain and fatigue, which in turn produce voice symptoms that are unattractive, interfere with communication, and can give a false impression of you.

A strained or tired voice can be hoarse, lack sufficient volume (and conviction), and often may have changes in pitch. Worst of all, a tired voice can elicit similar reactions from listeners. If a speaker sounds tired, the audience feels tired. If a speaker's voice sounds strained, you can see strain in the audience too — restlessness, inattention, even irritation, a "let's get this over with" reaction.

If your occupation requires you to talk a great deal, make a conscious effort to cut down on your talking during times when you don't need to speak when you are by yourself, during meals, and away from work.

The parts of the body that produce voice are largely muscle. We use muscles to take in breath and to control letting it out. Muscles in the larynx and vocal cords produce the sounds of language. As with any other muscles, prolonged use tires them. So in speaking, as in other athletic situations, give yourself a break during your breaks.

All of the chapters in this book are designed to help you use each element of voice production — breathing, phonation, and resonance — in a completely natural manner to lessen strain and fatigue.

Throat Clearing. When you clear your throat, the vocal cords rub tightly together as outgoing air violently passes between them. Over time, this can cause them to become irritated. The irritated cords then exude more mucous to protect themselves. When we feel the presence of this mucous, we clear the throat again to get rid of it, and the problem is aggravated.

Some of us also clear our throats when we are ill at ease or as a way of getting attention. Often, it is a kind of announcement that we are about to speak, and reflects our anxiety over how our first words will sound. In such cases, and they are very common, throat clearing is more of a habit than a way of getting rid of mucous on the vocal cords. It can be annoying for those listening to us. Worse than that, it can irritate the vocal cords enough to cause hoarseness.

For whatever reason, real or imagined, we do it, throat clearing should be a rare event. Instead, we recommend that you learn to *sniff-swallow*. If you feel that there is mucous in your throat, take an exaggerated and sudden sniff. This sudden inhalation will often dislodge any mucous on your vocal cords, which you can then swallow. (The normal person swallows quarts of throat mucous every day.)

Another technique for avoiding throat clearing is the *silent cough*. If you cough in a light but sudden whisper, this too will often dislodge vocal cord mucous, which can then be swallowed.

These tips are probably all you need if you have a throat-clearing habit, and we did not feel it was necessary to devote a chapter to this problem, even though it is a common one. One last word. If you do find it necessary to clear your throat from time to time, do it gently, not explosively. The kinder you are to your vocal cords, the kinder they will be to you over the years.

Throat Focus. Some people sound as if their voices come from deep down in their throats. Such a low throat focus often produces a voice pitch that is too low and a voice that is not loud enough. People who use a low voice focus often complain of losing their voices or of becoming hoarse after a lot of speaking. People who use an excessively high voice focus sound very nasal — and complaints are apt to come from people who have to listen to them.

With a normal focus, the voice sounds as if it is coming from the middle of the mouth, perhaps on the upper surface of the tongue. With this more vertical focus, you can usually use your voice all day long without developing any voice problems. As you listen to people who use their voices a lot — entertainers, actors, announcers, public speakers of all kinds — pay attention to where their voices seem to be coming from. These are people whose livelihood depends on good speaking habits; they cannot afford to develop voice problems. Almost certainly you will hear that most of them focus their voices in the middle of their mouths.

We will look at voice focus in more detail in Chapter 8, Is Your Voice in Focus?, and give you exercises for focusing your voice in the middle of your mouth.

Posture Problems. It may surprise many of you, but poor sitting and standing posture not only makes a bad visual impression, but can markedly interfere with producing a good voice, too. A typical poor sitting posture is the slouch: shoulders forward, abdomen protruded, and chin down. A slouched posture often results in a weak, ineffective, hoarse voice. Such a position makes it difficult for the body to take in the air it needs for good speech. Try it. Try taking in a breath while slouched. Then try taking in a breath while sitting tall, with your back firmly against the back of your chair and your shoulders back. In the latter position, you should feel a deeper inspiration of air that makes it possible to complete your phrases and sentences with adequate volume and a natural-sounding voice. People with sedentary jobs, in particular, need to watch their posture. They can often improve the sound of their voices by keeping in mind the command: Sit tall.

A good standing posture, standing tall, is also important to a good voice. The standing slouch is just as common as the sitting slouch, and the results for speaking are the same. There is, however, no need for a stiff, military stance. All you have to do is keep your body erect but relaxed. A good standing posture can be practiced with your back to a wall. Your heels, buttocks, and shoulder blades should touch the wall, along with the back of your head.

Two bits of imagery can also help. First, imagine that the back top of your head is hanging by a rope from the ceiling. This will put your head at the right angle with your chin neither too high or too low. Second, imagine that you have a large tail that you bring forward between your legs. This will help tilt your pelvis forward a bit, which in turn tucks in the abdomen.

These simple suggestions will help you not only sound better, but look better as well. If, however, you feel that you have a persistent posture problem that interferes with developing a good voice, you might want to consult a physiatrist (see Chapter 16) or a physical therapist. For most of us, however, the best posture for speaking is as easy as remembering what was said about sitting and standing tall.

Stressful Situations. All of the poor voice practices just discussed are commonly aggravated, or even initiated, by stress. Stress causes us to make unusual demands on our vocal equipment.

As we saw in the previous chapter, stress on the voice can come from things such as pollution, infections, smoking, and dietary practices. It can also stem from anxiety in our work, social, or recreational activities.

Anxiety reactions to stress affect our voices in two ways. They can cause us to tax our voices because we need to speak longer, louder, or with more intensity than usual. Or anxiety may cause us to speak in a voice that is not our natural voice.

We are all familiar with the voice symptoms of anxiety: the dry throat and mouth, shortness of breath, changes in pitch, all the things we associate with the term *stage fright.* In Chapter 10, Keeping Your Natural Voice Under Stress, we list 20 voice symptoms related to stress and show you techniques for overcoming them.

It is important to remember, however, that we are all "on stage" frequently in the course of our normal work and social lives. There are always times when you are called on to do something that is not routine, to give good or bad news or crucial information to those you work for or who work for you. In addition, many of us voluntarily subject ourselves to stressful situations in our recreations — in team sports, amateur or semi-professional singing or acting, even in informal social situations that suddenly turn formal when we are asked to say a few words or to offer or respond to a toast.

It is not possible, or perhaps even desirable, to eliminate all stress from our lives. It is possible, however, to minimize or eliminate stress symptoms from your voice when you feel the need to do so. To take some liberties with Rudyard Kipling's famous poem, "If you can keep your voice when all about you are losing theirs . . . " then you probably have used the techniques we describe in Chapter 11.

Misinformation. Many of us have received bad information about how voice is made, and why our voices sound the way they do. Some of us are chronically short of breath when we speak, because we learned somewhere that to get in adequate breath we need to work at it or to use diaphragmatic breathing. Or we have been told that our voice sounds best at the lowest pitch we can produce. Or that a loud voice makes us seem more confident, a soft voice more appealing. Virtually any of the problems discussed earlier in this chapter can be caused or aggravated by bad information about voice production, which can make it difficult or impossible for you to remedy them.

However, the most common bit of misinformation we have about our voice is this: Our voice is something we are born with, and whether it is pleasing to us or others, there is nothing we can do to change it. That is a very unfortunate bit of misinformation for the roughly 60 million Americans who have voice problems. The good news is that it is untrue. Most of us with voice problems have *made* our voices sound the way they do. We have learned bad voice habits and have persisted in using them.

What has been learned can be unlearned, and new voice practices can be developed that will give you a pleasing, natural voice. That is the essential message of this book. The following chapters will help you to identify specific voice problems and give you specific exercises to correct them. By replacing misinformation with good information, you will be able to find and use your natural voice.

CHAPTER **5**

To Breathe or Not To Breathe

"Breathing for speech is a natural process, as automatic as your heartbeat or blinking."

Many people seem to have all the breath they need when they speak. But others seem to run out of air and struggle to finish what they say. Robert was a case where running out of air almost meant running out of gas in an otherwise accelerating career.

In his early 30s, Robert's life had started to take off. Not only was he getting new responsibilities and promotions at the insurance firm that employed him, but increasingly he was also being asked to take on civic duties in the community where he lived.

Conscientious as always, Robert began to devote new attention to self-improvement, taking pains with his clothes and grooming and signing up for night classes. Because now he was asked to speak to groups, too, Robert thought it would be a good idea to get some experience in public speaking, and he joined the local chapter of a national speakers' organization. There he had his first serious setback. While he had a lot to say about business and community affairs, his speaking voice was a handicap, not a help, in saying it.

Listeners had a hard time understanding Robert because he was a "fader." His sentences started out clear and strong enough, but his voice soon faded away and people kept asking, "What did he say?" After a while, they lost interest. Some were irritated. By the end of his sentences, Robert sometimes was whispering.

When he came to us for help, I needed only to go to one of his speaking engagements to hear what the problem was. Robert often spoke as many as 30 words on one breath. It was too many. He was literally running out of air before he finished a sentence.

We demonstrated to him that all he needed to do was pause every 15 words or so. When he paused he took in a new breath without effort. By cutting down the number of words per breath, his voice was loud enough all the way through whatever he was saying. With some practice, Robert's serious setback soon turned out to be only a minor stumbling block in his rising career.

To Breathe or Not To Breathe

The miracle of breathing is that it is all done for us automatically from the moment we are born. When we need air for any kind of exertion, we automatically take in more and larger breaths. When we sleep, we don't need to instruct or monitor our breathing mechanism; it keeps working steadily and slowly.

All speech, and singing, is produced by the outgoing breath stream making the vocal cords vibrate. Breathing for speech is accomplished by a quick inspiration (so fast we are unaware of it), followed by a prolonged expiration. The voice is powered by the strength of the outgoing breath.

We usually take in more breath than we need to use for speaking. Most of us therefore have ample air for speech, and experience little or no breathing strain while talking. All we have to do is think about what we want to say and begin saying it.

Yet many people who have normal breathing mechanisms, free of disease, find themselves short of breath when they speak. In some cases the problem may be caused by simple anxiety, which can make breathing more rapid and shallower. If you think some of your breathing problems during speech come from anxiety and nervousness, in addition to reading this chapter you should look carefully at Chapters 10 and 11 on stress and stage fright to learn how to help your voice in such situations.

For many other people the problem is that they do not use their normal breathing mechanisms correctly when speaking. They usually fall into one of three categories.

- *The Athletes.* Instead of allowing breath to renew itself automatically, athletes try to *make* it work. They may raise their shoulders and gasp audibly (remember Billy Joe from Chapter 2?), keeping their diaphragms contracted. They may resemble a fish out of water, but they are just human beings, like you and me, running out of air.

- *The Gamblers.* The gambler doesn't take in enough air on a breath. He is in such a hurry to say something (perhaps because he is afraid of losing his listeners' attention) that he just grabs a quick, shallow breath and rushes on pell mell, gambling that he will have enough air to finish what he is saying.
- *The Spendthrifts.* These people may take in ample air with each breath, but then they carry on as if that breath will last forever, no matter how much they say. These are the people, like Robert, who habitually try to say too many words on one breath.

What all of these familiar types have in common is that they do not allow their breathing mechanisms to function naturally for them. Indeed, most of the time they behave as if breathing were an *obstacle* to speech, instead of the very thing that makes it possible. The gambler and the spendthrift seem annoyed at having to pause and take a breath, while the athlete seems to look at breathing as a series of hurdles he has to get over to say what he wants to say. And all of them are proving that they do a lot worse job trying to *make* breathing while speaking than just letting it occur more naturally.

The body has a lot of vital processes that are completely automatic, from blinking to heartbeat, and breathing is one of them. You don't have to consciously direct your blinking to keep the surface of your eyes moist or your heartbeat to keep blood pumping through your body. With breathing for speech, all you have to do is learn how to breathe (or relearn, since you were born knowing how) as naturally and easily when you speak as you do in the other activities of your life. The big difference for speech is that it requires a quick inspiration followed by a prolonged expiration, whereas for most of our other daily activities, inspiration and expiration are more nearly equal.

Breathing problems in speech can become habitual. They will get worse unless the person who has them takes steps to correct them. It isn't hard. In the tests and exercises that follow we speak of *breath control,* but what you will actually be discovering is natural control over breathing: the right amount of breath, the right amount of words you can say on a breath, and how to do this easily, without effort or strain.

THE BREATH CONTROL TEST

You will need a stopwatch or a watch or clock with a second hand to take this test. After taking in a slightly larger than normal breath, measure the seconds you sustain your expiration for each of the following tasks.

1. Take in a breath and then make a hissing sound: *sssss*. Sustain it as long as you can. After the first time, try prolonging the sound a few more times. Take the longest time value and enter your score here: _____ seconds.

2. Take in a breath and then count as far as you can while you exhale. After the first time, try a few more times to count farther. Time each attempt. Take your longest time and enter your score here: _____ seconds.

Scoring the Breath Control Test

1. Prolonging the *s*. In general, larger people with larger rib cages can hold on to an expiration longer than smaller people. Accordingly, there are different "normal" values for prolonging the *s*, depending on the age and size of the speaker.

Children ages 7 through 10 should be able to sustain an *s* for 8 seconds.

Children ages 11 through 15 should be able to prolong an *s* for 12 seconds.

Women 16 and older should be able to sustain an *s* for 15 seconds.

Men 16 and older should be able to prolong an *s* for at least 20 seconds.

If you cannot achieve these times, you may need practice on breath control.

2. Counting as far as you can. Different people count at different rates of speed, so for purposes of this test we will measure the number of *seconds* you can keep counting. The more words you say, the more breath you need, so try to count at a moderate rate.

Children under 10 years old should be able to keep counting for 6 seconds on one breath.

Children ages 10 through 15 should be able to count for 8 seconds.

Women should be able to count continuously for 10 seconds.

Men should be able to count continuously for 12 seconds.

If you cannot achieve these times, you may need practice on breath control.

Remember, The Breath Control Test is only a rough screening of how adequate your breath control is. After reading this far in the chapter, you probably already know whether or not you have a breath control problem. If you do, you will want to try some of the suggestions for breath control that follow.

THE BREATH CONTROL PROGRAM

The four steps presented here are designed to help you rediscover the breath control that you were born with. One way we will do this is to try to extend your outer limits of breath control. Once you have learned to do that, you can comfortably cut back from those limits so that you always have ample breath for a good, natural voice with minimum effort.

Breathing as a Continuous Motion

As your chest becomes bigger by active muscle action, the air comes in (inspiration). As the chest gets smaller, primarily from muscle relaxation, the air goes out (expiration). From the point of view of producing voice, however, it is important not to view inspiration and expiration as distinctively different events. Ideally, they are one continuous motion.

Two simple exercises in coordinating breathing with walking and talking will help you get a feel for inspiration and expiration as one continuous motion.

1. Take in a breath slowly as you walk five steps. As your leg swings into the sixth step, begin humming for the next five steps. Now keep walking, breathing in slowly for five steps, humming for the next five steps, and so on. Practice until this comes easily for you.

2. Take in a breath slowly as you walk five steps. As your leg swings into the sixth step, begin counting 1-2-3-4-5. Count one number for each step. Now repeat the walking cycle, inhaling slowly for five steps, then counting 1 through 5 for the next five steps. Keep practicing until this comes easily for you.

Improving Your Expiratory Control

Now that you have developed a feel for inspiration and expiration as one continuous motion, you may also need some practice in prolonging expiration.

In the real world of talking, inspiration is very quick, a fraction of a second, while expiration-talking may last for several seconds. Your results in The Breath Control Test have shown you whether your expiration is adequate for your age and sex. If it is not, the following exercises will help you improve it. As you do them, avoid taking in "the big breath," and don't raise your shoulders or push down. Just take in an easy breath and begin.

1. Using a stopwatch, or a watch or clock with a second hand, see how many seconds you can produce each of these sounds.

SSSSSS   ZZZZZZ   EEEEEE   AAAAAH

2. Use the number of seconds as your baseline measure. If, for example, you can prolong the *sssss* for 8 seconds, 8 seconds is your baseline.

3. Now try prolonging the sounds past your baselines. With practice, you can exceed your baselines by perhaps 2 seconds a day. Keep practicing until you can prolong the sounds for about 15 seconds.

These exercises will help you develop ample air reserves for what you want to say.

Matching Target Models

The average speaker is able to time with amazing accuracy the right amount of breath for what he or she wants to say. For most of us this process is completely automatic. We have enough breath, and we have it with no special effort, no audible gasps or body contortions or observable strain.

One of the best ways to achieve this easy, natural breathing is by practicing on target model sentences. For example, have someone say a seven-word sentence, such as

THE STOCK MARKET GOES UP AND DOWN.

You will need a partner to help you with this exercise. The partner reads the sentence aloud. You listen. Then the partner points to you to repeat it. Ask the partner to vary the time between when he reads the sentence and when he points at you to repeat it. The idea is for you to repeat the sentence as soon as possible, with no thought about taking in a breath. When you get the cue, say the sentence quickly and in an easy, relaxed manner on one breath.

Here are some short sentences for you to practice on:

HOW ARE YOU?

HELLO, HOW ARE YOU?

OPEN THE BROWN DOOR.

MONEY, MONEY, LOTS OF MONEY.

AN OLD WOMAN OWNED THE NEW LAND.

ANNIE LIKED HER HOME ON THE RANGE.

HAND OVER THE FOUR MISSING ORANGES.

THE OLD MAN ON THE BUS READ THE PAPER.

SHE WENT OFF HER DIET WHEN SHE DINED OUT.

THE WOMEN IN THE OFFICE HAD THEIR OWN PARTY.

Once you can repeat the target model sentence on cue, without any special breathing effort, practice reading aloud at your own pace, without any signal, using any reading material you wish.

On The Breath Control Test, how many seconds were you able to count on one expiration? Repeating sentences on cue, and oral reading on one breath, need be only a fraction of that time. The most air most of us would ever need while speaking should be used up in less than 5 seconds.

After a few weeks of practicing matching target models, you will find that you can say more words per breath with very little effort. You will also learn how many words you can comfortably say on a breath. With that information as part of your speaking behavior, you are now ready to learn to pause.

Renewing Breath by Learning to Pause

The magic word for breath control in speaking is *pause*. It is that simple. So many of us work so hard to breathe while we speak, when all we have to do is pause to renew our breath. When we pause the muscles for inspiration contract, our chest gets bigger, we draw in needed breath, and we can continue talking comfortably. The pause should become part of your continuous motion of breathing, a reflexive part, one that you are not even aware of.

The timing of the pause should not compete with the verbal message. It doesn't need to if we practice finding the right places to pause.

Our grammar school teachers taught us to write in complete sentences, and we should speak in complete sentences too. But that does not mean one complete sentence on each breath. Many sentences are too long for that.

Any place in an utterance that contains natural punctuation, such as a period, semicolon, or comma, is a good place to pause. A good place to pause is also when you are trying to recall a word or an idea, or when you are thinking of what to say next. A poor place for a pause would be between an adjective and a noun [She's a pretty (PAUSE) girl], or between a verb and an adverb [He really (PAUSE) tried].

Using your tape recorder, practice reading the following paragraphs, pausing where indicated in the text.

HARVEY'S WIFE, *pause* JOANNE, *pause* FOUND OUT ONE DAY THAT SHE WAS ACTUALLY HARVEY'S FIFTH WIFE, *pause* THAT HE HAD A SERIES OF MARRIAGES *pause* ONE RIGHT AFTER THE OTHER. *pause* EACH OF THE PRECEDING WIVES HAD NO KNOWLEDGE *pause* THAT HARVEY WAS ALREADY MARRIED, *pause* AND CERTAINLY NOT *pause* "SEVERAL TIMES BEFORE." *pause* BY TALKING WITH OTHER WOMEN AT HER HEALTH CLUB, *pause* JOANNE FOUND OUT THE NAMES AND AD-DRESSES OF THE OTHER WIVES *pause* TO WHOM HARRY WAS STILL MARRIED. *pause* JOANNE GATHERED ALL OF THE WIVES TOGETHER ONE NIGHT. *pause* EACH WOMAN THOUGHT THAT HARVEY WAS A TRAVELING SALESMAN, *pause* WHICH WAS WHY HE ONLY CAME *pause* "HOME" ONCE A WEEK. *pause* TOGETHER, *pause* THEY PLANNED A HOMECOMING THAT HARVEY WOULD NEVER FORGET.

IN THE NEW AGE OF SCIENCE AND SPACE, *pause* IMPROVED EDUCATION IS ESSENTIAL TO GIVE NEW MEANING *pause* TO OUR NATIONAL PURPOSE AND POWER. *pause* IN THE LAST 20 YEARS, *pause* MANKIND HAS ACQUIRED MORE SCIENTIFIC INFORMATION *pause* THAN IN ALL OF PREVIOUS HISTORY. *pause* NINETY PERCENT OF ALL THE SCIENTISTS THAT EVER LIVED *pause* ARE ALIVE AND WORKING TODAY. *pause* VAST STRETCHES OF THE UNKNOWN ARE BEING EXPLORED EVERY DAY. *pause* FOR MILITARY, MEDICAL, COMMERCIAL, *pause* AND OTHER REASONS. *pause* AND FINALLY, *pause* THE TWISTING

COURSE OF THE COLD WAR *pause* REQUIRES A CITIZENRY THAT UNDERSTAND OUR PRINCPLES AND PROBLEMS. *pause* IT REQUIRES SKILLED MANPOWER *pause* AND BRAINPOWER *pause* TO MATCH THE POWER OF TOTALITARIAN DISCIPLINE. *pause* IT REQUIRES A SCIENTIFIC EFFORT, *pause* WHICH DEMONSTRATES THE SUPERIORITY OF FREEDOM. *pause* AND IT REQUIRES AN ELECTORATE IN EVERY STATE *pause* WITH SUFFICIENTLY BROAD HORIZONS AND SUFFICIENT MATURITY AND JUDGMENT *pause* TO GUIDE THIS NATION SAFELY THROUGH WHATEVER LIES AHEAD.[1]

The commas, periods, and stress places in the above paragraphs provide natural places to pause. During each pause, your breath should have been renewed naturally, with no special effort on your part.

Now listen to the recording of your reading. Are those natural places for you to pause? Do you need to pause more often or less often?

Try pausing in different places in the text than the ones I marked. Now listen to how the pauses work for your breath control, and for the sense of the material. You may want to ask someone else to listen to your recording and see how they evaluate you for ease of speaking and for the sense of what you are saying.

Practice with paragraphs from books and magazines, too. Mark them for pauses. Then read paragraphs you haven't marked to see if you are developing a natural feel for when you need to pause.

Pausing easily transfers to the real world of talking. One of the first things you will find out is that your listeners don't run away when you pause. In fact, if anything, the pause will make you a more effective speaker. Good pauses make your meaning clearer. Good pauses give a natural emphasis to those parts of what you are saying that you want to stress. And the pause, so brief that it is hardly noticeable, gives you the continuous breath supply you need for speech.

Too little air, too many words, too much effort. Any of these symptoms in speech are clear signs that you are not allowing your natural breathing to function. Because breathing for speech can become as automatic your heartbeat or blinking, correcting your problem is not a matter of learning something difficult and new. By following the suggestions in The Breath Control Program you will learn to do what you were born knowing how to do: breathe easily enough to speak in a normal, natural voice.

---

[1]Excerpted from a speech to Congress by President John F. Kennedy, January 29, 1963.

CHAPTER 6

Loud Enough or Too Loud?

"Your voice has a loudness control too."

Your Loudness Control

Radio, television, and stereo sets have a loudness control. We can adjust their volume to a comfortable level so that music or speech is intelligible, yet not so loud or so faint that it is annoying. When it comes to our voices, however, many of us fail to realize that we need to use a loudness control in just as discriminating a manner. We need to adjust the loudness of our voices for different speaking situations.

An overly loud voice can signal that the speaker is aggressive and unfriendly, or brash, boorish, or insensitive. A voice that is too soft can suggest that the speaker is shy, indecisive, has low self-esteem, or doesn't really care to communicate.

Like other voice characteristics discussed in this book, the loudness of your voice may be telling on you, and it may tell the wrong story. Loudness conveys the strength of our feelings, our level of confidence, and whether we are anxious or hostile or comfortable with those around us. We use loudness to project our voices across distance, yet our loudness level also conveys the emotional distance we want with other people. A voice that is too loud keeps people at arm's length. A voice that is too soft can signal that you don't want to bridge the gap between other people and yourself.

We need to vary our level of loudness for different physical distances between us and our listeners, to accommodate for different levels of background noise, and to convey different emotions. The problem is that many people use the same level of loudness all the time. They do this for a variety of reasons.

Take the case of Ed, the 55-year-old Dean of a School of Business Administration at a major university. Visitors to his office were quickly turned off by a voice so loud that he seemed aggressive. As one colleague put it, "He's always giving a speech instead of just talking with you."

In fact, as part of his work, Ed did give a lot of speeches to business groups. And, over the years, he had begun to emulate the speaking style of the hard-charging executives and entrepreneurs he had met and admired.

Although such a voice might have been appropriate for his lecture audiences, students and faculty reacted differently. His colleagues thought him authoritarian and a man who liked to talk more than listen. Students were so intimidated by him that they dreaded visits to his office, and often came away not remembering what he said.

When Ed finally came to us, we heard at once that the voice he used in our offices was not the voice that was giving him his problem. What we heard was the moderate voice of a man who had realized that he had a voice problem and wanted to do something about it.

Which was Ed's real voice, the one that caused his colleagues to refer to him (he had learned only recently) as "Thundering Ed," or the softer voice of the man asking us for help?

It was both. Ed hadn't realized that the loudness level appropriate for one speaking situation and one kind of audience might not be appropriate elsewhere — that, in fact, most of the people he spoke with weren't an "audience" at all.

Ed confessed to us that he had come to like his hard-charging voice. He liked the image of himself that he thought it projected. Without giving it much more thought than that, he had adopted it as his customary voice.

We were able to show him exercises to help him find his volume control, so that he could adapt his loudness for different settings, yet still command attention and carry conviction. "Thundering Ed" still inspires them on the lecture circuit, but colleagues, students, and friends are now far more comfortable with his "voice of moderation."

Like Ed, all of us can learn to use the volume control for our voices. Relatively early in life, we all learned to use the loudness level that got things done for us, that produced the reaction we wanted. For example, when we are with a loved one we use a soft voice. When we want the kids to turn down their stereo, we often find that a loud voice is necessary. In some business or professional situations, we may need to speak a little more loudly to add authority to our voices. But some people either are uncertain what volume level is appropriate or, for other reasons, fall back on using the same level of volume. It is these habitual loudness levels that cause problems.

That was the case with Linda, a 25-year-old secretary. Being a secretary was not her first choice of career. She had studied to be a teacher and even had her teaching credential. But in her student-teaching days she discovered that her voice was not loud enough for students only halfway back in the classroom to hear, unless she really "forced" her voice. When she did, her voice would not last through the day. She would be physically exhausted, and her throat would be raw.

Instead of trying to change her voice ("I didn't know I could. I thought it was something I was born with," she told us), Linda decided to change her career. However, the problem that had plagued her in the classroom followed her to the large medical office where she worked next.

Although she could be understood well on the telephone, like many soft-spoken people can, Linda had difficulty being understood by the team of doctors she worked with and by their patients. She was always being asked to "speak up," or to repeat things she had said.

When Linda came to us for help, we discovered that the voice she was "born with" was in fact a voice that she had acquired because it seemed to please other people. Hers was a little-girl voice, one that early in her life her parents and friends had found cute. Later, her dates in high school and college not only found it cute, but sexy. Linda's voice was light and breathy and had so little volume that people had to lean closer to hear what she was saying.

A voice evaluation showed that Linda's breath inhalation for talking was no greater than what she used just sitting in front of her word processor. As a result, besides speaking almost inaudibly at times, she commonly ran out of breath when she spoke, and had the habit of leaving sentences incomplete. Listeners not only had trouble understanding her, they thought she didn't have much to say — or, at any rate, didn't care to communicate it.

We were able to help Linda, first of all, by showing her that her "cute" voice was not her natural voice, but a very artificial one. Once she realized that, we were able to show her techniques, which are described later in this chapter, to take in larger breaths and to pause more often when she spoke. With more available breath, she could speak louder without strain. With adequate pauses in her speech, she could renew her breath and complete all of her sentences with plenty of volume.

Linda discovered that speaking loudly enough to be easily understood made her much more effective and appreciated in her work. It was also far from a drawback socially. Linda was just as attractive as ever. Only now people paid attention to her for *what* she said and not for the dismaying way she once said it.

Appropriate Loudness

In noisy environments, most of us adjust our loudness level automatically. In a disco, on a jet plane, or talking to someone using a power mower, we raise our voices until we can be heard. Similarly, in a church, a hospital, or near a room where someone is sleeping, we lower our voices so that they are not disturbing.

The noise levels in our immediate environment are very obvious clues to the loudness levels we need to use. Many people, like Ed and Linda, have trouble adjusting loudness in more ordinary circumstances. Ed would not dream of dressing inappropriately for a lecture, nor Linda for her day at the office. But neither exercised the same sensitivity for their voices.

To help you gain awareness of how loudly you customarily speak, we have developed a Loudness Rating Scale. It has five voice levels:

1. **Whisper.** We use no voice at all as we whisper to someone near us.
2. **Soft Voice.** The kind of voice that would not wake someone sleeping nearby.
3. **Conversational Voice.** This is a loudness level that matches that of the people we are talking with.
4. **Loud Voice.** This is the voice we use in front of a group (without using a microphone), or when we want to command attention.
5. **Yelling.** We use this when we are angry, or demand to be heard, or in sports, as players or spectators.

Keep these loudness ratings in mind as you take the simple test that follows. It will give you a clearer idea of the relative loudness of your voice and is the first step for gaining control of your voice volume, whatever circumstances you find yourself in.

THE VOICE LOUDNESS TEST

Using a book like this, it is not possible to precisely measure the intensity of your voice. Such a measurement requires equipment like a sound level meter. Also, as we have discussed, your voice loudness can, and should, change from situation to situation.

But by following the two steps of this test, you can tell whether or not you need to alter your customary loudness. The latter part of this chapter will give you exercises for changing and controlling your level of loudness.

1. Gather around a table with a few friends or colleagues willing to help you with the test. (They might find the results interesting for their own voices.) In the center of the table place a tape recorder, and record 20 minutes or so of spontaneous discussion in which you actively participate. Now listen to the playback.

- Is the loudness of your voice similar to that of the other participants? If it is, your loudness in this situation seems adequate, and on the Loudness Rating Scale your voice would probably be a Level 3, conversational voice.
- If the loudness of your voice is different from that of the others, would you rate yourself as a Level 2 (soft voice) or a Level 4 (loud voice)? We assume that you neither yelled nor whispered. If you were consistently louder than the others, you need to learn to soften your voice. If you were consistently softer, you need to increase your loudness.

Both kinds of exercises will be given later. But first complete Step 2.

2. The purpose of this step is to assess how loudly you speak customarily, not just in a special test situation. As accurately as you can, respond *true* or *false* to the statements below.

I vary the loudness of my voice as I speak.	＿＿
My voice loudness is appropriate for most speaking situations.	＿＿
People seldom ask me to repeat what I have said.	＿＿
People seldom ask me to speak more softly.	＿＿
People seldom ask me to speak more loudly.	＿＿
Overall, I am pleased with my voice loudness.	＿＿

If you answered *true* to each statement, your voice loudness is probably adequate, although you may want to check your rating with that of some of your friends. If one or more of the statements do not seem to apply to you, you probably need to work on the loudness level of your voice.

What we are concerned with is a *customary* level of loudness that is inappropriately loud or soft. If the above tests suggest that you need to decrease or increase your level of loudness, the exercises that follow will be of help.

EXERCISES FOR CHANGING YOUR VOICE LOUDNESS

Decreasing Voice Loudness

First of all, it is important to realize that a common cause of an overly loud voice is hearing loss. Hard-of-hearing speakers generally use a louder voice, and are often slow to realize that they have a hearing problem. If there is any question of hearing loss, have your hearing checked by an audiologist or otolaryngologist (ear-nose-throat doctor).

If hearing loss is not the cause of your speaking too loudly, the first step in correcting the problem is to become aware that the problem exists. The Voice Loudness Test has helped you do this. Now, a little practice with the following exercises can help you to develop a softer voice.

1. Review the five loudness levels in the Loudness Rating Scale (whisper, soft voice, conversational voice, loud voice, and yelling). See if you can produce these levels in various sequences. We will omit practice in yelling because it is hard on the larynx — and the ears of anyone listening to you. Try saying HELLO, HOW ARE YOU? at four loudness levels, varying the order in which they occur, as illustrated below.

soft–loud–whisper–conversation
loud–whisper–conversation–soft
whisper–soft–conversation–loud
conversation–whisper–loud–soft
soft–conversation–whisper–loud

Now try counting from 1 to 10 using the different loudness levels as above. To fix the differences clearly in your mind, it may be helpful to use your tape recorder. You will soon realize that the loud voice level requires a lot more effort. It is far easier to use the whisper or soft voice.

This exercise helps you develop your own "loudness control" so that, as you do with your radio, television, or stereo, you can adjust your voice volume so that it is intelligible and comfortable for you and your listeners.

2. Now that you can produce different loudness levels, try using the soft voice level in some conversational situations. You may be surprised how often it is an appropriate voice, even though most of the time outside your home Level 3 (conversational voice) is what you want to use. Level 4 (loud voice) should only be used in situations where much volume is necessary for others to hear you, for instance, in noisy environments or before large groups. What you are developing with this exercise is sensitivity to the appropriate loudness level for each speaking situation. The best rule is: Never use a loudness level greater than necessary.

3. Also develop your sensitivity to the varying noise levels around you, at home, in your car, at work, and in recreational settings. Before you speak, take a second to register the noise level in your immediate environment. After you have done this for awhile, you will automatically adjust your voice loudness level so that you can always be heard above the background noise.

Increasing Voice Loudness

We need to devote a little more space to these exercises than the previous ones because speaking too softly seems to be a more common problem than speaking too loudly. This is particularly the case among women because so many of them have been conditioned to think that a soft voice is more feminine and attractive.

Once the Voice Loudness Test has made you aware that you need to speak louder in certain situations, the following practice steps will help you use a louder voice.

1. Develop your sensitivity to situations where others have trouble understanding you. Where do you most often hear reactions such as "What?" or "Would you please say that again?" These are obvious clues that you need to speak louder. But there are less obvious clues too, in facial expressions and body language. If listeners look bored, inattentive, or fidget when you talk, it may not be because of *what* you are saying, but *how* you are saying it. Nothing tries people's patience more than a speaker who does not make himself heard. A speaker who is too loud may irritate, or even affront, listeners, but one who speaks too softly can forfeit his listener's attention completely.

2. Check your articulation. Are you a mumbler? Some people habitually fail to articulate sounds such as *t, d, sh, ch, k, g, f,* and *v.* Articulation and loudness usually go hand in hand. If you do not articulate clearly, no amount of volume will help you be understood. On the other hand, well-articulated speech at too low a volume is still indistinct speech. Listen to a recording of your own speech. Do you make the sounds listed above as clearly as they can be made? If this is particularly difficult for you, you might want to consult a speech-language pathologist (see Chapter 16) for some help in this area.

3. An easy way to make your voice louder is to take in a slightly larger than normal breath. As you probably discovered in experimenting with the levels of the Loudness Rating Scale, speaking louder not only requires more effort, it takes more air. Try it. Try saying, "HELLO, HOW ARE YOU?" taking in varying amounts of air before you speak. Practice this until you automatically take in the right amount of air for the loudness you want.

4. One way to be sure you have enough air for an adequate loudness level is to cut down on the total number of words you say on one breath. Use a tape recorder to check the number of words you customarily say on a breath. If lack of air causes your voice to become softer, cut the number of words from, say, 15 words to 10 words on each breath. In other words, *pause* more often. Use your tape recorder and experiment until you find the number of words between pauses that consistently gives you adequate volume for your speech.

5. Elevating your voice pitch by about one note can also make your voice easier to hear. Level 2 (soft voice) can often sound like Level 3 (conversational voice) when you raise your pitch a note. In Chapter 7 we will show you ways to elevate your voice pitch. For many of you who have problems being heard in conversational or work situations, raising your pitch level may be all you need to do.

6. Practice reading aloud, combining what we have just said about pausing more often and elevating your pitch level a note. Tape-record your reading. First, read with your old, customary voice. Then use the breathing and pitch elevation tips for the second reading. Listen to the playback. You should sound louder. If you do not, steps 7, 8, 9, and 10, which follow, should help you.

7. There is also a lifting technique that you can practice to produce a louder voice. Once you experience producing this louder voice, you will no longer need to use the lifting exercise. Here is how it works:

> Sit in a chair with your arms extended below the seat on each side. Count aloud from 1 to 10. As you count, reach under the seat and try to lift the chair off the floor. You won't be able to get the chair off the floor, of course, but the muscular exertion used should increase your breath force, tighten your vocal cords, and result in a louder voice.

> Repeat the counting and lifting action while tape recording the exercise. On playback, can you hear a louder voice while trying to lift? If you did, go back and practice exercises 3, 4, and 5. Now that you have found a louder voice, these exercises will help you control it when you want to.

8. Open your mouth a bit more when you speak. Many people who mumble or speak too softly do so because they do not open their mouths enough when they speak. This may be a problem of yours.

Look at yourself in a mirror when you speak. Do you open your mouth, or do you speak through clenched teeth and almost closed lips?

Try opening your mouth more when you speak. Allow your lips to shape the words and syllables. You would be unable to speak distinctly if someone put his hand over your mouth when you tried to talk. Keeping your mouth closed is like putting your hand over your mouth.

9. This step will require someone else to help you. You will also need to wear earphones connected to some kind of music source such as your cassette player, a radio, or a stereo.

Put on your headset and listen to some music at a low level of volume.

Instruct the other person to change the volume of the music higher or lower while you read aloud into a tape recorder.

After reading aloud for two or three minutes, stop and listen to the tape. You will be amazed at how loud and clear your voice can sound when you speak with loud music in your ears.

Once you have taped your louder voice, you can use it as a model for practice, just as you did with the lifting exercise. Your memory of your louder voice will be good enough so that you usually will be able to match it without needing the loud noise or music in the background. Reinforce your control by going back and practicing exercises 3, 4, and 5.

10. If, after all of the above, you still have a problem making your voice a bit louder, turn to Chapter 8, Is Your Voice in Focus? In that chapter we talk about bringing the focus of your voice out of your throat and placing it in the general area of the mouth. A well-focused voice, coming from the front of the mouth, usually produces a louder voice.

Now that you have learned how to adjust and use the "loudness control" of your voice in various situations, you should find that you can always speak at a loudness level where you are heard and understood — but never louder than is necessary. An appropriate level of loudness is one of the keys to your natural voice.

CHAPTER **7**

The Well-Aimed Pitch

"You can really throw your listeners a curve with an inappropriately pitched voice."

Pitch is a key element of our voice "fingerprint," one of the characteristics that makes our voices distinctively our own. Even without seeing a person, it helps tell us immediately whether the speaker is male or female, and roughly what his or her age is.

From pitch, we can gather other specific information, too. While there are normal pitch ranges for each sex and age group, there is considerable variation in habitual pitch level from individual to individual. Moreover, when we speak, most of us vary our pitch in a distinctive manner, stressing some words and not others. (We do this with loudness too.) This pattern of rising and falling pitches we call voice inflection.

Both our habitual pitch level and our pattern of inflection help pinpoint who we are and what kind of person we are. As is true with other elements of voice, often we have acquired these pitch characteristics sometime in our past and take them for granted as part of our voice. But a voice that is pitched too high can make an otherwise masculine man sound feminine. A woman's voice that is pitched too high can make her sound like a person who is not to be taken seriously. For either sex, a voice pitched lower than it should be can strain the vocal equipment and affect intelligibility. And all of us know how tiring and irritating a monotonous voice without inflections can be. In short, a mispitched voice can send an inaccurate or unfavorable message about us and also damage the voice.

The latter was the case with Sammy, 25 years old and a new biology teacher at a suburban high school. He felt he looked too young for his age, and that because he did he had discipline problems with his classes and was not as effective a teacher as he knew he could be.

Sammy's reaction was to do a number of things to seem older, like wearing dark, conservative suits and discarding his contact lenses in favor of glasses. He even grew a mustache.

He also tried speaking in as low a voice as he could to sound more mature. The result of that, however, was hoarseness and sometimes loss of voice toward the end of the school day. The problem became so severe that eventually he came to our voice clinic. We found that he was speaking all day at the bottom of his pitch range, an octave below low G on a piano, while his tested range would go from that note to the piano's middle E. We advised him to raise his regular speaking pitch up three notes. (Most of us should use a pitch two to three notes above our lowest note.) We gave him practice exercises to do this, and within a week the hoarseness and fatigue disappeared.

We will soon show you how to find your own natural pitch level, and how to raise and lower your pitch if you need to. However, the point about Sammy is that his voice strain was caused by constantly speaking below his natural pitch level.

Many people have the opposite problem: speaking above their natural pitch level. This is sometimes found among girls or women who imagine that a higher pitch will make them sound more feminine. But if this is not the normal pitch for their voices, the result can be the same voice strain that Sammy experienced.

No one should speak at the same pitch level all of the time. Rather, pitch should constantly vary with inflections up and down. However, there does appear to be one pitch level that we hear most of the time in a speaking voice and identify as the person's habitual pitch. There also appears to be a natural pitch level where the voice is produced with the least amount of muscular effort. This easy voice can usually be heard in the easily produced "uhm huh" voice described in earlier chapters.

We usually find the natural pitch several notes above the bottom of our pitch range. The natural pitch often includes more than one note, sometimes adding the note above it and the note below it. The human voice does not cling to one speaking note. While we can identify one habitual pitch in the voice, it is important to remember that there is continuous fluctuation above and below this pitch.

Let us look first at what the normal pitch levels are for men and women of various age groups. Then we will give you tests to establish whether your habitual speaking pitch is approximately where it should be and give you some exercises to raise or lower it if it is not. Finally, we will make some recommendations for gaining control of pitch so that your speech has good pitch inflection.

Finding Your Natural Pitch Level

In our voice clinics we have electronic instruments that quickly tell us what pitch level a person is using. We measure pitch range and habitual pitch by measuring the number of vibrations per second of an individual's vocal cords. The frequency of vibration per second is known as the Hertz (Hz) value. The Hz value can also be expressed in the notes of the musical scale as played on a conventional 88-key piano.

Although many of you will not have access to a piano, for purposes of illustration, we show in Figure 7-1 where the natural pitches of the voice fall in terms of musical notes.

You will notice that the keyboard is divided into octaves, each whole octave (there are two partial ones) consisting of the notes C-D-E-F-G-A-B, ignoring the sharps and flats. The lowest note on the keyboard is A, the highest is C8, and middle C, midway between the bass and treble clefs, is called C4.

Using this illustration, we show the typical pitch levels for certain ages and sex. The pitch levels shown are normal, natural pitch levels, the kind of pitch we often use when we agree with someone by saying "uhm huh." As you can see, the speaking voice pitches of adult men and women fall only in the range of octaves 2, 3, and 4.

Both the normal pitch level and overall pitch range (from the lowest to the highest note you can reach) can vary from individual to individual. Some of us have naturally lower or higher pitched voices than others.

The basic pitch level and range of the voice is determined by the physical size of the larynx. But we ourselves change our voice pitch as we speak, or sing, by changing the tension of the vocal cords. When they are contracted and thick, we produce lower pitches. When they are stretched, the tension on the cord increases, and we produce higher pitches. In normal conversation, at our natural pitch level, the vocal cords need very little stretching. Consequently, our voice sounds relaxed and resonant. This is the goal we need to achieve.

TWO SELF-TESTS FOR FINDING YOUR NATURAL PITCH LEVEL

There are two ways we can find out what our natural pitch level should be. A simple way that requires no musical knowledge is our first self-test, The "Uhm Huh" Voice Pitch Test. Our second pitch test, the Music-Assisted Voice Pitch Test requires some basic musical knowledge. We usually find that the "uhm huh" and the music-assisted tests identify

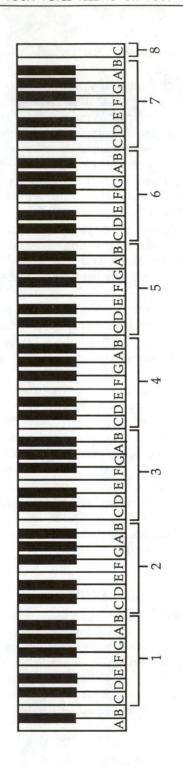
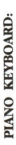

PIANO KEYBOARD:

Sex and Age and Natural Pitch Level	HZ	Musical Note
Babies, 10 months old	400 Hz	near G4
Boys and girls, age 9	260 Hz	near C4
Women, age 21	195 Hz	near G3
Women, age 51	175 Hz	near F3
Men, age 21	130 Hz	near C3
Men, age 51	110 Hz	Near A2

FIGURE 7-1. Typical speaking pitch levels for age and sex.

the same natural pitch level, but the music-assisted test identifies the pitch more precisely by musical note.

The "Uhm Huh" Voice Pitch Test

You may or may not be using a natural pitch level. One way to find out is to take this simple test.

1. Use your tape recorder. Read aloud a paragraph from the newspaper and record it. Listen closely to the pitch of your voice on playback. Does your pitch level sound too high or too low? Does your pitch seem to vary up and down as it should?
2. Make a recording of conversation with several of your friends (all of the same sex). Listen to the playback. Does your voice pitch sound similar to the voices of the other men or women? If your pitch sounds lower or higher, you may have some realistic concern about your voice pitch level.
3. Record yourself saying "uhm huh." It is best to do this by reading a question aloud before saying it. Read the question and then stop. And then say "uhm huh" as if you were responding to a question. For example, read aloud

   DO YOU BELIEVE THAT THE AMERICAN PUBLIC WANTS SPACE EXPLORATION?

   Now answer, "uhm huh." Repeat this several times.
4. More often than not, the "uhm huh" has been said at a pitch that is very near your natural pitch. Listen to the pitch level of your "uhm huh" several times. See if you can match it by saying "one, one, one" at the same pitch level. Listen to your tape playback. Does your saying "one, one, one" show a pitch level that you feel needs to be higher or lower in pitch? How does it vary from the pitch you used in saying "uhm huh" and in reading the sentence out loud?
5. Say other questions aloud, and follow each by "uhm huh." Listen carefully to the playback. If you feel that your pitch level and your pitch inflection is not a problem for you, you can skip reading the balance of this chapter.

If you feel you want to raise or lower your habitual pitch based on your experience with the "uhm huh" testing, you might turn to the "Uhm

Huh" Pitch Practice exercises given later in this chapter. If you want to work now on pitch variability, go to Practice in Varying Your Pitch.

The Music-Assisted Voice Pitch Test

For the reader who has a good musical ear and access to some kind of pitch-generating instrument (piano, guitar, pitch pipe), this self-test is much more precise in determining habitual and natural pitch levels than the "uhm huh" self-test.

This test requires a cassette recorder and an instrument that can produce a single note. Your task will be to play a note, or have someone else play it, and see if you can vocally match it. If you have a good ear, you can do the test by yourself. If you have difficulty finding the notes or matching the pitches with your voice, ask someone to help you.

1. Select a note easily produced by persons your age and sex. Play this note (see keyboard in Figure 7–1) as your model:

   Teenage girls, play G3
   Teenage boys, play D3
   Adult women, play F3
   Adult men, play B2

2. Match the model note by saying "eee" at that same note. Then sing down one note at a time, saying "eee" until you produce the lowest "eee" you can make. For example, if you started at B2, the adult male model note, you would sing down, saying "eee," voicing the notes B2, A2, G2, and F2. Your lowest note would be F2.

3. Our natural pitch levels are usually a few notes above our lowest note. Start with your lowest note and say "eee." Go up one note at a time for just two more notes. This could be very close to your natural pitch level, a note that you can produce with very little effort.

4. Now sing up three notes, saying "eee" above your lowest note. This note, too, could be a natural pitch level for you. Most of us have one or two notes that we produce easily. Remember, the natural pitch level for speaking is always a few notes (two or three) higher than the lowest note you can sing. But, most important, stay off the bottom of your pitch range.

Now that you know where your natural pitch ought to be, find out what your habitual pitch is. Tape-record some conversational speech and oral reading. Listen carefully to the playback. Introduce your natural pitch level (the pitch you just determined) and compare it with your recording. You might ask someone else to help you make this judgment. Is your habitual pitch at the same level as your natural pitch? If it is, you probably do not have to work on changing pitch.

If you want to change your habitual pitch to more closely match your natural pitch, the exercies that follow will help you.

PRACTICE IN PRODUCING
YOUR NATURAL SPEAKING PITCH

Learning to relax the vocal tract can help you find your natural pitch and maintain it once you have found it. With less tension, the vocal cords produce the pitch level that is natural for them. Here are two techniques that are helpful for getting this relaxation.

The Yawn-Sigh Method

Taking in a bigger breath on a yawn, and letting it out on a sigh, immediately relaxes the mouth and throat. Practice prolonging sounds as you sigh. First yawn (with no voice) and then sigh out the air with light voice. Your pitch level on the sigh will be close to your natural pitch. Practice extending the sigh using these five sounds:

AAAAAAAH   AAAAAAARM   AAAAAAALL   HAM   HARM

The sigh-induced voice is particularly good practice for those who need to lower their voice pitch.

The Chewing Method

Many people with pitch problems don't open their mouths as wide as they should, and often speak through clenched teeth. This is a tense way to speak. The chewing approach will help develop an open, relaxed mouth and throat. After practice in speaking while chewing, your voice will produce a pitch very near your natural pitch level. This exercise may not be pretty to look at, but it is fun to do — and it works.

1. Practice chewing in front of a mirror. Open your mouth at least two fingers wide between your front teeth. Move your jaw and tongue up and down and exaggerate the movement of your mouth.
2. Add light voice while you chew. This will produce a monotonous *yahm-yahm-yahm* kind of sound.
3. Now practice saying these nonsense words as you chew:

    MOONAMONGA   ALAMETERAH   CUCALAMONGA

    Prolong the words as you say them until they sound almost like a chant. The voice you produce while doing this should be near the natural pitch level that you are trying to achieve.

These exercises are useful for reminding yourself what your natural pitch level sounds like and also will help you to relax your mouth and throat so that you can produce it.

We now need to consider some specific exercises for either raising or lowering your pitch level.

Practice in Lowering Your Pitch

On either of the two previous tests, if you found that you need to lower your pitch level, the practice steps below can help you. The first practice session uses the "uhm huh" as your reference voice. The second section uses actual musical pitch as your practice guide.

Using the "Uhm Huh" as Your Practice Guide

1. Use the steps you used in the "uhm huh" test to establish your practice "uhm huh." This "uhm huh" is a lower pitch than you generally use, otherwise you wouldn't be trying to lower your habitual pitch to this new, lower level. As we practice on other words, we will always come back to your "uhm huh" as your reference sound.
2. Record your "uhm huh" and repeat it several times on tape. Listen to the playback. Can you reproduce it just as it sounds on the tape? If not, practice with your recorder until you can always produce the "uhm huh" the same way. Once you can comfortably produce the "uhm huh," go ahead to the next practice step.
3. Practice saying the "uhm huh" followed immediately by repeating these words:

```
ONE     ONE     ONE
MAN     MAN     MAN
MANY    MANY    MANY
ONE-TWO-THREE-FOUR-FIVE
ONE-TWO-THREE-FOUR-FIVE-SIX-SEVEN-EIGHT-NINE-TEN
```

Record this practice step. Listen to the playback. Does your pitch level on the words stay on the same level as on the "uhm huh"? Repeat it so that all the words are on the same "uhm huh" pitch.

4. Read aloud from a magazine or newspaper. About every 10 words, say "uhm huh" and try to maintain that kind of pitch level for the total reading. Record your oral reading practice. Did you stay at the lower pitch?

Using a Musical Pitch as Your Practice Guide

1. The easiest way to lower your pitch, if you have a good ear, is to play the note that represents your natural pitch. Use this now as your practice note. See if you can match it with your own voice pitch.

Prolong the pitch with an extended "ah."

Practice reading aloud in a monotone using this new pitch.

Make a recording of your voice using the new pitch in both reading and conversation. Keep your voice at a monotone, using the new pitch for all words. Listen to the playback. If you are satisfied that you kept the lower pitch throughout the reading, go on to the next step. If keeping the new pitch is difficult, repeat the first two steps.

2. Speak in your higher voice, the one that you found was your habitual pitch. Take a word like *man* and prolong saying it at that pitch level for about three seconds. It will sound like *maaaaaan*. Now practice saying *man*, prolonging the length of the word, as you descend down the musical scale to the lowest note you can produce. Record your practice effort as you say:

MAN (your habitual pitch)
> MAN
>> MAN ***
>>> MAN
>>>> MAN

Now listen to the playback carefully. Did the words sound better — more resonant, louder, and more relaxed — at one of the pitches? If so, this could well be your natural pitch level. Practice saying the word, two or three notes from the bottom. Was the best sounding word the one that is marked ***? Often your best, or natural, pitch level is two notes above your lowest note.

3. Keep practicing the lower pitch level until you find it comfortable. It may take a few days of practice.

Practice in Raising Your Pitch

A voice with too low a pitch level usually lacks carrying power, projection, and full resonance. If, on the previous tests, you found that you needed to raise your pitch, some of these suggestions will help you.

Using the "Uhm-Huh" as Your Practice Guide

You found on testing that your habitual pitch was lower than the pitch you use when you say "uhm huh." Use your tape recorder for these practice suggestions and listen carefully to the playback.

1. Speak at your regular pitch level (the one you found was too low). Read a sentence or two from a newspaper, suddenly stop, and say "uhm huh." Listen to the playback. Is the "uhm huh" slightly higher in pitch? Now read again but try to keep it at the higher "uhm huh" level. If you were able to do this, try to do more reading at the higher level.
2. Go back to your regular, lower voice. Say "one, one, one" at that lower level. Now see if you can go "one, one, one" up the scale from your regular voice, like this:

>>>> ONE
>>> ONE
>> ONE ***
> ONE
ONE (your low, regular voice)

Listen to the third word (marked ***) closely. This might be the higher pitch you are looking for. See if you can match this higher pitch with other words.

3. Practice saying words in a monotone at the higher pitch level, the one marked ***. Do some monotone reading at the same higher pitch level.

You have now found a higher pitch level, perhaps at or near your natural pitch level. Try practice speaking at this level.

Using a Musical Pitch as Your Practice Guide

1. The easiest way to raise your habitual pitch is to play the note that you tested as your natural pitch on a piano or a pitch pipe. Attempt to match it with your own voice.

Prolong the natural pitch with an extended "ah."

Practice reading aloud in a monotone voice with the new pitch.

Record the new, higher pitch level. First, record your prolonged "ah" and then the monotone reading. Listen to the playback. See if you can match (imitate) your own recorded models.

2. Elevating your pitch a note or two is not difficult. It is more natural to raise your speaking pitch a bit more than it is to lower it because you have many more notes available above your habitual pitch than below it.

3. Practice saying these sentences, raising your pitch at the end of the sentence:

HOW ARE YOU TODAY?

HOW LONG IS THE STORY?

DID YOU POINT YOUR FINGER?

WHERE ARE YOU GOING TO GO NOW?

WHEN WILL THE IRANIANS EVER BE HAPPY?

Practice using the higher pitch by reading aloud in a monotone for a few minutes, several times a day. Practice using the higher pitch in conversation with someone you know well. With some practice, the higher pitch can be part of your new natural voice.

Practice in Varying Your Pitch

Pitch inflection is part of the melody of a language, and makes most languages distinct from one another. Chinese, for example, is a tonal language, with great sweeps in pitch. Some of those pitch changes add different meanings for the same word root. Although some Spanish and Portuguese and French words look alike when written, it is not just different pronunciation that makes them sound different but varying pitch inflections, too. The importance of inflection is even clearer in dialects of the same language. Southerners in the United States, for example, not only pronounce words differently than people in New England do, but the way they stress the language is markedly different.

The melody of inflection in the speech of individuals is also part of their distinctive signature when they speak. In English, certain pitch inflections have come to signal certain character traits. For instance, as we point out in later chapters on men and women's voices, pitch that drops at the end of phrases and sentences (characteristic of men) connotes authority and sureness, while pitch that rises (characteristic of some women) connotes unsureness and shyness.

When we had university students write down words they thought best described the meaning of pitch inflections of well-known people, the low-pitch inflections of William Buckley were seen as "authoritative, aggressive, in command, decisive, controlling." The rising inflections of a Truman Capote were viewed as "effeminate, ambivalent, indecisive, questioning, unsure." In the case of Lyndon Johnson, who lacked good pitch variability, the students wrote, "loss of affect, boredom, no emotionality, fatigued."

Overall, inflections are what give distinctive personality and liveliness to our speech. There is nothing more boring, and eventually irritating, than listening to someone who speaks in a monotone. The normal voice should go up and down around one's natural pitch.

Because lack of inflection, or misplaced speech inflections, can send negative signals about us, most of us can benefit from becoming more critically aware of our habitual pattern of speech inflection. The way to do this is, of course, to listen carefully to our own voices and the voices of those around us.

On your cassette recorder, tape your own voice and the voices of some of the people you hear on television or radio. When you play them back, write down, as our university students did, your impressions of what the voice inflections convey to you. Try to pay attention exclusively to the inflections, rather than other speech characteristics. Now compare your ratings of your own voice with those of the others you have recorded. If, overall, you rate the others higher or lower than yourself, can you tell what differences in inflection patterns were crucial in your judgments? What are they doing with their inflections that you don't want to do, or would like to do?

We will show you now some exercises for gaining control over your voice inflections so that you can achieve the pattern you want.

Practice in Rising and Falling Inflections

1. Using the words *well, yes?,* and *no?* practice rising inflections as shown below.

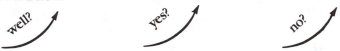

2. Using the words *go, why,* and *no* practice falling inflections as shown below.

3. Using the words, *no, when,* and *yes* practice double inflections, a rising pitch that drops off to a falling pitch. This kind of pitch bending in a single syllable word seems, as you will hear, to convey sarcasm, uncertainty, or double meaning.

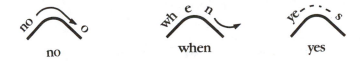

| no | when | yes |

4. You now should have heard how changing the inflection of a word can give that word a special meaning. (This can also be done to some extent by changing your loudness.) Actors and actresses of course have refined their talent for using changes in inflection to convey inner feelings. But all of us do this, consciously or unconsciously, in our daily lives. To gain conscious control over this process, practice the following exercises. Using the word *now,* try to inflect the word so that it conveys each of the feelings listed.

anger	sad	hopeful	sickly
sarcastic	sexy	scared	happy
defeated	shy	thrilled	disgusted

After you have practiced this for awhile, record your efforts and ask another person to listen to the recording and write down what emotion he or she hears in your voice. Practice this until the word the other person writes down is the word for the emotion you wanted to convey.

5. Finally, you need some exercise in changing pitch inflections not just in single words but in the course of an entire sentence. Read aloud the sentences below, making the pitch changes that are indicated. The words and syllables level with the dash are at your normal pitch; the others are above or below it.

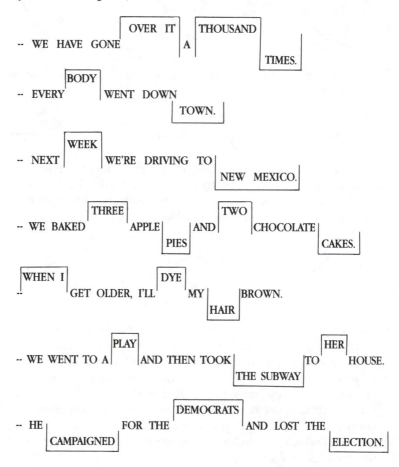

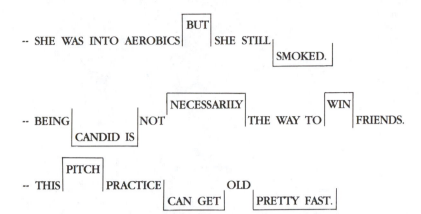

6. After you can read those sentences comfortably, without hesitating, record your reading. What kinds of meaning and emotion do you hear? Now try making different inflections, even on different words, and write down the different meanings and emotions you hear. You can also try this exercise with sentences of your own or sentences from magazines that you have marked for inflections. In a short time, you will begin to hear that the meaning of a word or a sentence can be dramatically changed with slight changes in inflections.

Pitch is like a facial expression conveyed purely by sound. Imagine saying any of the sentences you have been practicing accompanied by a smile, a frown, a sneer, or a twinkle in your eye. Try this in front of a mirror and you will see that you have profoundly changed the meaning of what you are saying by your accompanying expression.

Pitch changes have the same effect on your speech. A high-pitched voice, a low-pitched one, and a distinctive pattern of inflections all contribute, almost as much as the dictionary definition of the words you are saying, to the meaning and emotional content of your speech.

Changing your pitch level, if it needs to be changed, and gaining control over your pitch inflections, can greatly improve the way you sound and prevent serious misunderstandings. With proper use of pitch, you can say what you mean and be perceived as always meaning what you say.

CHAPTER 8

Is Your Voice in Focus?

"What you want to avoid is a voice that sounds as if it's stuck in your throat, or falling off the tip of your tongue."

Vocal coaches say that to produce good voice the vocal tract needs to be in focus, just as you need good camera focus for a clear photograph.

Of all the voice characteristics that we talk about in this book, focus is the most difficult to describe. It is easy to understand what we mean when we say someone speaks without enough breath, or too high or low in pitch, or too loudly. But what do we mean by good voice focus? We mean a voice that sounds as if it is coming from the middle of the mouth, just above the surface of the tongue. The drawing on the next page, Figure 8-1, will help you visualize this, a voice focused at the X where lines A and B, the horizontal and vertical planes of the vocal tract, cross.

Another way to make the concept of focus clear is by describing what bad, or poor, focus is. Look at the illustration. If your voice is produced from a point too high or too low on the vertical line, B, it will have poor vertical focus. Similarly, if your voice is produced too far forward or too far back on the horizontal line, A, it will have poor horizontal focus. Now let's "listen" to a couple of cases where focus was used poorly.

Twenty-seven-year-old Rick and his partner Robbie started a wine shop in a fashionable shopping center of a large city. Robbie mostly took care of the back-room chores, the ordering of inventory, and the books. Rick was the front man with, both partners thought, a gift for dealing with customers.

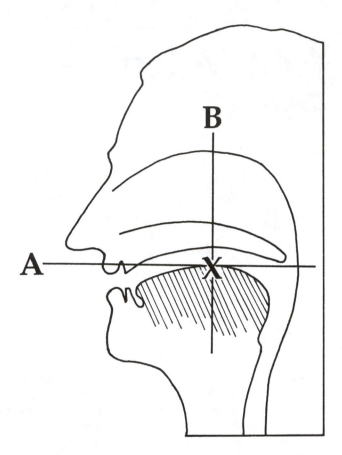

FIGURE 8-1. Voice focus. Normal voice focus (✗) is at the intersection of line A (horizontal focus) and line B (vertical focus).

But the two men had been friends for so long that they took a lot about one another for granted — including the way they spoke. Neither reflected on the fact that, while Rick had an engaging personality, he had a high pitched voice, with a thin front focus, and even a slight frontal lisp, which often results from a voice produced near the tip of the tongue.

They realized they had a problem, however, when it became obvious that when Rick was out front customers didn't linger and didn't buy. But when Robbie filled in at the counter they made sales. As both partners had staked their life savings on the venture, they took the problem seriously. Rick came to us for voice therapy.

Our goal was to develop exercises that encouraged Rick to use a more posterior carriage of the tongue. We will show you those exercises later on. They worked for him. As his tongue came back to a more neutral position, the high, thin voice began to disappear, and so did the severity of his lisp. With this improved horizontal focus, and much practice, Rick developed a nice-sounding baritone voice — and the store a steady clientele.

A case of someone with a problem of vertical focus was Carl, a successful manufacturer's representative in his early 40s. His voice was produced from deep in his throat. At the same time he always tried to speak at the bottom of his pitch range, which compounded the problem.

As with so many types of voice misuse, hoarseness was the symptom that finally got Carl's attention. His hoarseness was so bad that sometimes he could scarcely speak at the end of the day.

When he came to us, our voice evaluation showed him to have a normal larynx, throat, and mouth. What he needed was to get his voice out of his throat and into his mouth, to develop a better vertical focus. He was able to do this in his first therapy session. He was a little more resistant to using a higher pitch. Like many men, Carl thought the lower his voice, the more macho he sounded. But when he listened to tape playbacks he realized how much better, and how much clearer, he sounded with the combination of higher focus and higher pitch. After six weeks of therapy, and much self-practice, his hoarseness was totally gone, and whenever Carl needed voice, which was often in his line of work, he had a good one.

Finding the Focus and Balance of the Natural Voice

Let us now look more closely at what makes horizontal and what makes vertical focus. Your voice originates in your larynx. As outgoing air from your lungs passes between your two vocal cords, it sets them in vibration. This vibratory sound, you will recall from Chapter 2, is called *phonation,* or voice.

As sound waves, the vibrations then travel from the larynx into your resonating cavities, your throat, nose, and mouth. The particular shapes, and the changing openings, of these resonating cavities are what help give you your distinctive voice. Our unique, basic sound depends to a great extent on how wide open our mouth is, the relative openness of our throat, and the position of our tongue.

Where the tongue is in the mouth contributes to what we call horizontal focus, and strongly affects our voice resonance. A normal voice has a balanced horizontal focus; the tongue is neither too far forward nor too far back when we speak. When the tongue is excessively forward, as shown in Figure 8-2, we produce the kind of voice that was such a prob-

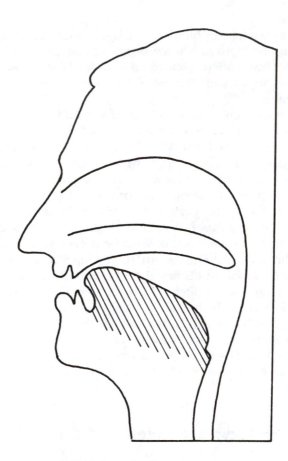

FIGURE 8-2. Front voice focus.

lem for Rick in our first example: weak, thin, and, in his case, with a distinct lisp.

A posterior carriage of the tongue, as seen in Figure 8-3, is the opposite problem. In extreme cases, those who use it sound like the television character Alf, or, for those of you with good memories, like Edgar Bergen's Mortimer Snerd.

In both cases, resonance can suffer. The best horizontal focus, and the best voice, comes from a tongue carried in a neutral setting, in the middle of the mouth.

Vertical focus, on the other hand, doesn't involve tongue placement, but where the voice is produced in relation to the tongue. Some voices sound locked low in the throat, as was the case with Carl. Other voices sound focused above the tongue, high in the nose. In fact, there are so

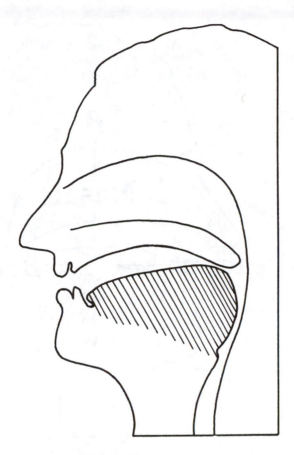

FIGURE 8-3. Back voice focus.

many people with nasal voices that we will devote a separate chapter, the following one, to the problem. Normal, good voice focus sounds as if the voice bounces off the surface of the tongue in the middle of the mouth, as shown in Figure 8–4.

Your mental image of "placing your voice" in this position is as important to keeping a good vertical focus as the position of your tongue is to horizontal focus.

TEST FOR VOICE FOCUS

Most people have no voice focus problem. If, however, you find that you have a focus problem (front-back-low [throat]-high [nasal]) after tak-

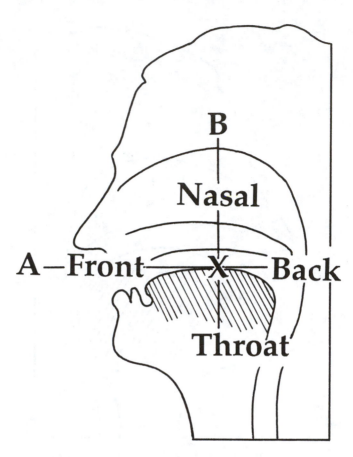

FIGURE 8-4. Voice focus sites. X = normal.

ing this brief test, the exercises and suggestions that follow the test can help you develop a more normal sounding voice focus.

You will need your tape recorder. You will also need the list of 100 voice descriptors that you studied in Chapter 1. The list has been reproduced here as Table 8-1 for your use on the Test for Voice Focus. Although you can complete the test wholly on your own, it would be helpful to have a friend help you make some judgments about how your voice sounds.

1. Make a recording reading aloud this passage:

TO SUCCEED IN LIFE ONE HAS TO BELIEVE IN ONE'S SELF. IT IS VERY EASY TO LET OBSTACLES IN LIFE BECOME ACHIEVE-

TABLE 8-1. 100 Word-Descriptors for Voice

____ 1. abrasive	____ 35. flat	____ 68. pingy
____ 2. affected	____ 36. feminine	____ 69. pleasing
____ 3. baby	____ 37. fluttering	____ 70. poor
____ 4. bad	____ 38. forced	____ 71. powerful
____ 5. beautiful	____ 39. glassy	____ 72. quivering
____ 6. bell-like	____ 40. golden	____ 73. relaxed
____ 7. blanched	____ 41. good	____ 74. resonant
____ 8. bleary	____ 42. gravelly	____ 75. rich
____ 9. breathy	____ 43. harmonious	____ 76. ringing
____ 10. bright	____ 44. harsh	____ 77. rough
____ 11. brilliant	____ 45. heady	____ 78. round
____ 12. bubbly	____ 46. heavy	____ 79. scratchy
____ 13. burnished	____ 47. high	____ 80. sexy
____ 14. buzzy	____ 48. hoarse	____ 81. shallow
____ 15. cello-like	____ 49. hollow	____ 82. sharp
____ 16. chesty	____ 50. husky	____ 83. silken
____ 17. clangy	____ 51. immature	____ 84. silvery
____ 18. clear	____ 52. insecure	____ 85. smooth
____ 19. coarse	____ 53. intimidating	____ 86. sophisticated
____ 20. confident	____ 54. light	____ 87. stentorian
____ 21. constricted	____ 55. lovely	____ 88. strident
____ 22. cool	____ 56. low	____ 89. sultry
____ 23. covered	____ 57. macho	____ 90. thin
____ 24. crude	____ 58. masculine	____ 91. throaty
____ 25. cutting	____ 59. mature	____ 92. tight
____ 26. dark	____ 60. mellow	____ 93. timid
____ 27. deep	____ 61. melodious	____ 94. velvety
____ 28. dead	____ 62. metallic	____ 95. warm
____ 29. dry	____ 63. monotone	____ 96. wavering
____ 30. dull	____ 64. nasal	____ 97. wet
____ 31. effeminate	____ 65. open	____ 98. whining
____ 32. effervescent	____ 66. painted	____ 99. whiskey
____ 33. edgy	____ 67. pinched	____ 100. white
____ 34. fearful		

MENT BARRIERS. THIS CAN MAKE US END UP FOCUSING ON WHAT WE CANNOT DO. IT WOULD BE FAR BETTER TO FOCUS ON WHAT WE CAN DO, OR AS LEE IACOCCA MIGHT HAVE SAID, "THERE IS NO GREATER TONIC FOR BELIEVING IN ONESELF THAN HAVING SUCCESS."

2. Now ask a friend to help you judge your voice focus. Show him or her the list of 100 word-descriptors for voice. Once you have reviewed the list together, tell your friend to listen to your recording of the paragraph and select the 10 words from the list that best describe your voice. You, also, will select 10 descriptive words from the list at the same time.

3. Now compare your list of 10 words with your friend's list. If you have normal focus, there is usually less agreement between you and someone else than if you have a focus problem. If you have a focus problem, you will usually have *three or more words* that you and your friend have agreed on.

4. Using the words that you both agree on, see if you find each word listed in the columns below. We have listed the words that typically describe a focus problem under the four out-of-focus headings below:

Front	*Back*	*Throat*	*Nasal*
baby	bell-like	bubbly	clangy
brilliant	burnished	chesty	cutting
constricted	cello-like	deep	harsh
effeminate	covered	forced	heady
feminine	dark	golden	high
immature	flat	gravelly	metallic
light	hollow	heavy	nasal
shallow	open	hoarse	pinched
thin	resonant	husky	pingy
timid	silken	low	ringing
white	silvery	macho	sharp
	stentorian	masculine	strident
	velvety	rough	whining
		sultry	
		throaty	
		whiskey	

5. If you find three or more of the words that you and your friend agreed on in the same column, you probably have that particular focus problem. If there are only one or two words in one column or most

words are scattered across the columns, you probably do not have an obvious focus problem.

If you feel that you have a voice focus problem but were unable to identify it clearly (you did not have three or more words in the same column), you may wish to consult a speech pathologist (see Chapter 16). If you found that your voice may have a front or back or low or high focus, practicing the appropriate exercises that follow may help you.

EXERCISES FOR CHANGING YOUR VOICE FOCUS

Correcting Front (Anterior) Focus

Excessive front focus comes from carrying the tongue too far forward. Front-of-the-mouth focus can, however, be corrected with some practice on the following exercises.

1. Practice making the isolated *k* and *g* sounds:

KUH	KUH	KAH	KAH
GUH	GUH	GAH	GAH

The consonants *k* and *g* are made with the tip of the tongue down and the back of the tongue arched up against the posterior palate. They are back-in-the-mouth sounds. Just saying them in a slightly exaggerated manner can completely eliminate the front-of-the-mouth sound of your voice.

2. Practice prolonging the vowels in each of these *k* and *g* sounding words. You should feel the back focus of the voice as you say them.

KEEP	KEY	KOOK	COKE	COOK	COD
COMB	CORN	CAR	CULT	COME	GO
GOAT	GOD	GUARD	GUILT	GULCH	GOT GUM

3. Now practice reading aloud the *k* and *g* sentences below, keeping the voice back. This time record your reading on your tape recorder.

CANDY CANES CRUMBLED AT CHRISTMAS.
THE CONSERVATION COMMITTEE WAS CANDID.

CAROLE HAD A CALORIE COUNTER ON THE CANNISTER.
COUNTRY COUSINS CAME TO THE CORN SHOW.
CARL FOUND A CARBON COPY OF THE CABIN CRUISER.
GREAT GRANDMOTHER GROUND THE CORN
FROM THE BIG LEAGUES HE WENT INTO BIG GOVERNMENT.
HE GRABBED UP THE GREEN GRAPES FROM THE GRAPE BAG.
THE ALLIGATOR FEARED THE BEAGLE GUIDE DOG.
THE GOVERNOR'S SHAG RUG IS NO LONGER GOLDEN.

4. Listen to the playback. By now your voice should have less anterior focus. If you can, read a few of the sentences in your old voice, then a few in your middle-of-the-mouth voice. Can you *feel* the difference? Can you *hear* the difference?

5. If the above steps have not helped you enough to develop a voice with less front focus, repeat all the steps *and* drop your pitch one note as you do the exercises. Lowering the voice one note may reduce front voice focus.

Correcting Back (Posterior) Focus

Because the tongue is so far back in the mouth, speakers with a back focus often lack clarity of speech articulation. The exercises to develop more front focus are the opposite of those for developing back focus, and are designed to bring the tongue farther forward. Try the following:

1. Say each of the words below in an abrupt *whisper* (do not use voice).

PEEP   PIPE   PEACH   PEAS   PEAT   PIE   PATCH

The *p* sound is made by pursing the lips, filling the cheeks with air, and suddenly releasing it.

THIS   THAT   THIN   THINK   THICK   THIGH   THATCH

The *th* sound is made by sticking the tongue out between the front teeth as you make the sound.

SEE   SAT   SIN   SINK   SICK   SIGH   SEAT

The *s* sound is made by placing the tip of the tongue behind the upper front teeth as you make the sound.

2. Now say each of the previous words, first in a whisper and then quickly with voice. Your voice should feel and sound more forward than back.

3. Elevate your voice pitch by one note and try reading the sentences below in the higher pitch. Record your reading.

TEACHERS EAT RIPE PEACHES AT THE BEACH.

PETE BOUGHT AN APPLE PIE AT THE BABY BAKERY.

THE THISTLES SPRANG UP BY THE PINE TREE FOREST.

THEY ATE PEACH AND RASPBERRY TARTS AT THE TABLE.

PEOPLE THAT BUY BIG AUTOMOBILES PAY MORE FOR FUEL.

THERE MUST BE FIVE OR SIX PEACH TREE STREETS.

PENNY TYPED ON THE BIG ELECTRIC TYPEWRITER.

THEY BOUGHT A WREATH OF ROSES FOR THE TEACHER.

STOCK PRICES WENT UP BEFORE WE SOLD OUR STOCKS.

THE PEOPLE SEEM TO WANT MORE SPACE EXPLORATION.

4. Listen to your recording of the sentences. When you recorded them you should have felt the words spoken in the front of the mouth. By now your voice should sound focused more in the mouth than in the back of your throat.

5. Select a paragraph or two from a book or magazine. Read it aloud in what you think is your new voice, with more front focus. Then, if you can, read it in your old way with back-in-the-throat focus. Can you feel the difference? Now read the material again, recording it, but this time read it once with what you think is front focus and then with what you think is back focus. You should be able to hear the difference on playback.

Correcting Throat Focus

The person with poor vertical focus, who appears to "speak in the throat," places unnecessary strain on the larynx. Correcting the problem requires a good mental image of where the voice is coming from, and specific focusing exercises to help you place it where you want.

1. Try saying "EAT A BITE OF PIE," back in your mouth, then deep in your throat, and then high in your nose. If you can make those focus changes with relative ease, you should be able to "lift" your voice to where it should be, toward the surface of the middle of your tongue.

2. Record your attempts to move your focus around like this, every now and then using your old, low-throat voice. You should hear a marked contrast between the balanced voice coming from the middle of the mouth and the low-throat voice. Practice using the balanced voice until it becomes habitual. If you cannot do this with relative ease, try the following steps.

3. Make a very nasal voice, placing your voice high up in your nasal cavities. This is only a temporary step to get your voice out of your throat. Now, in an exaggerated nasal voice, say:

MANY-MANY-MANY
MAN-OH-MAN-OH-MAN
MONEY-MONEY-MONEY
RING-RING-RING

As you say these words nasally, place your fingers on the bridge of your nose. You should be able to feel the vibrations of the nasal cartilages and bones as you speak. To further experience this high nasal focus, say the following phrases aloud:

MAN IN THE MOON
MANY MEN WANT MORE MONEY
ONE TIME ONLY
MORNING SUN IN THE MORNING

4. What you have been producing is a high nasal, vertical focus — higher than you want. But it brought your voice out of your throat. What you need to do now is to bring your voice to the target focus area that we showed you in Figure 8–4 on page 76. Think of the × area in that drawing as your own mouth. Try to say the following words with your voice focused at that ×.

RASPBERRY PATCH
PEACH TREE PLAZA
EAT A BITE OF PIE
ELECTRIC TYPEWRITER
BABY BAKERY

5. Record your reading of the exercises in steps 3 and 4 and listen to the playback. You should hear a sharp contrast between the two focus points, nasal and middle of the mouth. If you cannot hear the difference at first, repeat steps 3 and 4. Once you have heard the difference, try reading, and recording, the following passage with your voice placed at the X-focus site.

THERE ARE MANY SATELLITES CIRCLING THE EARTH. SOME HAVE BEEN PLACED IN ORBIT BY THE SPACE SHUTTLE WHILE OTHERS HAVE BEEN BLASTED INTO ORBIT BY LAUNCHED ROCKETS. EVENTUALLY, THE SATELLITES WILL BE SERVICED AT SPACE STATIONS WHICH WILL ALSO BE CIRCLING THE EARTH AT VARIOUS ORBITAL ALTITUDES.

Listen to the playback. Is your focus where it should be? If it is, you are well on your way to being able consistently to get your voice out of your throat.

6. Remember that a major part of good vertical focus depends on imagery. We cannot physically place the voice anywhere. But by focusing our minds on a physical site in the vocal tract we can produce a marked difference in the sound of our voice. Keep that picture of the X-focus site in Figure 8–4 in your mind. Summon it up before you speak. If you do this, speaking in the middle of your mouth on the surface of your tongue soon will become second nature to you.

7. Of course, good vertical focus requires a good ear as well as good imagery. Most of you probably have found that you used the imagery well and have got your voice out of your throat. You can hear the results on the playbacks of your recordings. But if, after going through these steps a second time, you still have a throat focus, you might want to contact a speech-language pathologist (see Chapter 16).

Correcting Nasal Focus

For those of you with a vertical focus problem in the nose, turn now to the following chapter.

Good imagery is important to your being able to locate and sustain good voice focus. And good voice focus is equally important to the voice image of yourself that you project.

With the concept of focus now in mind, think back to the voices of the famous people we talked about in Chapter 1. The best of the voices, in addition to other positive qualities, have excellent focus. It is a major part of what gives their voices clarity and assurance, and what enables them to project their voices with no sound or sign of effort.

Despite the improvements you have made so far in your breathing, loudness control, and pitch, you still require good focus to project your voice both naturally and attractively.

CHAPTER 9

Talking Through Your Nose

"Following your nose is good advice for finding a lot of things — but not your natural voice."

While a mildly nasal voice can be tolerated fairly well by most people who have to listen to it, excessive nasality often costs a speaker a lot in both business and social situations. A nasal voice is unattractive to begin with. It can become irritating if we have to listen to it for long.

Like many voice problems, nasality is something the speaker may be aware that he or she has to some extent, but may be unaware of just how bad it really sounds and, worst of all, may assume that nothing can be done about it anyway.

That was the case with Bernice who at 35 was a sales representative for a paper goods manufacturer in a major sales market. Bernice had always been in sales. She attributed the fact that she had changed jobs, and product lines, as often as she had to the nomadic habits of salespeople. But in fact there was another pattern to Bernice's job switching. She began each position with fair success, but then experienced a slow, steady erosion of customers. She would begin to have trouble scheduling appointments; more and more of her phone calls found her clients "busy," and they returned her calls less and less.

"Why doesn't anyone want to talk to me anymore?" she complained to her sales manager. In response, she got the best critique of her career. "Maybe the problem is that they don't want to *listen* to you," he said.

That was what brought Bernice to us. We heard her extreme hypernasality at once and suspected it was the source of her problem. Testing showed that the cause was not physical. Her mouth and throat were normal. She could close off her nose from her mouth when she wanted to. So we were quickly able to demonstrate to her that she had the physical capability to have normal resonance.

We then gave her some voice models, free of nasality, to imitate, and she could do it. We recorded the results, and compared them with the old voice that she had first brought to our office. Bernice was amazed. She knew that she spoke nasally, but she had never known how bad it sounded. In fact, she told us that, like a great many people even in this high-tech age, she had never heard a recording of her own voice.

A voice therapy program was started which enabled Bernice to make good oral resonance a normal, natural part of her speaking. In three months her voice was free of hypernasality. It turned out that Bernice had a very attractive natural voice to go with her naturally ingratiating personality. And her customers were happy both to talk to her and to listen to her.

Before we continue, we need to point out that Bernice's problem was one of *two* kinds of problems that people have with nasality. Her case was one of *hypernasality*, the familiar whining or twanging voice that seems locked up in the nose. Some people, although far fewer, have the opposite problem, *denasality*, where there is insufficient nasal resonance.

The causes, and treatment, of each type of problem are very different, and we will examine them in more detail in a moment. But first let's look at a case of denasality.

Howard, 36, was a first officer flying "right chair" for a major airline. Among flight crews, Howard was continually kidded about sounding most of the time as if he had a severe head cold. He spoke in a muffled voice that was hard to understand, lacked resonance for the three sounds in English that need it, the *m*, *n*, and *ng*, and compromised even some of his oral sounds.

Comments on his voice from air traffic controllers and passengers, however, were not kidding. For the former, not being able to understand Howard was serious. In the case of the passengers, it was frustrating, irritating, and, in the case of nervous passengers, sometimes alarming.

More often than with cases of hypernasality, denasality can stem from physical causes, such as large adenoids high in the throat that block the free passage of air and sound waves into the nose. People who have trouble breathing through their noses often turn out to have such a physical problem.

We found, however, that Howard's problem was functional, not physical. For whatever reasons, he carried his tongue so far back in his mouth that he shut off the passages to his nose. His voice resonanted more in his throat than in either his nose or mouth. Most of the time he also seemed to speak at the very bottom of his pitch range.

All of the things he had been doing to produce his back, muffled voice were corrected by voice therapy. He used the exercises presented in Chapter 8 for developing better oral focus. The pitch raising exercises shown in Chapter 7 helped him raise his speaking pitch a couple of notes. His denasality was further helped by following the exercises at the end of this chapter for reducing denasality. Howard's voice greatly improved, allowing him to give much clearer cockpit radio responses and clearer instructions to his passengers. He called recently to tell us that both his airline career and private life had improved greatly "since getting my voice out of my throat."

Let us look now at the causes of both hypernasality and denasality. Then we will give you tests for both kinds of problems and show you some exercises to correct them.

Hypernasality

Only the three nasal sounds, *m*, *n*, and *ng*, receive their primary resonance within the nose and nasal cavities. All the other sounds of English are diverted into the mouth where they get their primary resonance. The sounds of voice coming up from the vibrating vocal cords are diverted out of the mouth by the palate. In Figure 9-1 we see a line drawing of the palate-throat closing mechanism.

In this side view of the mouth we see the bony hard palate (A), the soft muscular soft palate (B), and the back wall of the throat or pharynx (C).

In Figure 9-2, we see the normal open palate. The soft palate (B) is relaxed and hanging down, allowing air flow and sound waves to travel into the nose. During normal speech, the soft palate continually lifts up and touches the throat wall near the point C in the drawing. This elevation of the soft palate shuts off the mouth from the nose, and diverts the sound waves from the vocal cords into the mouth. Thus voice resonance is in the mouth and throat, below the closure point B.

In normal voice, the closure point opens only for the nasal resonance of the sounds *m*, *n*, and *ng*. In cases of hypernasality, however, it remains open and all voice sounds are given a nasal resonance.

Hypernasality can have physical causes, among them a physically short palate, a cleft palate, or weakened palatal muscles. If you think your hypernasality has a physical cause, you should find sources for help among the specialists listed in Chapter 16.

In this book we are concerned with those of you whose hypernasality has a functional cause, as was the case with Bernice. The upcoming Tests for Nasality will help you determine if you have hypernasality, and if the problem can be eliminated with exercises or requires specialized professional treatment.

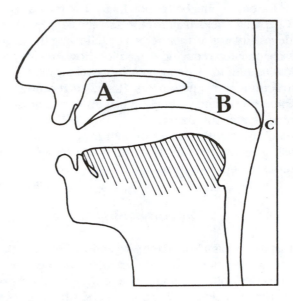

FIGURE 9-1. The normal closed palate-throat mechanism.

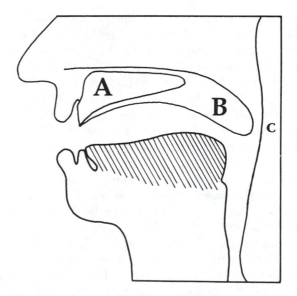

FIGURE 9-2. The normal open palate-throat mechanism.

Denasality

In denasality the sound waves of the voice cannot get into the nasal cavities to resonate for those *m, n,* and *ng* sounds, and in addition some of the vowel sounds and even the oral consonants can be impaired slightly. The resulting voice sounds like someone speaking with a head cold, and, as was the case with Howard, other people often have difficulty understanding what is said.

More often than not, denasality has a physical cause. In Figure 9-3, we show such a blockage. In this side view, we see excessive tissue (like adenoids and tonsils) in the area of the pharyngeal wall (C). Even though the soft palate (B) may be dropped and open, there is so much tissue between B and C that sound waves cannot get into the nasal cavities.

Some problems of denasality, however, do not have such a physical cause and can be helped with speech-voice exercises. Our Tests for Nasality will tell you if your resonance problem is denasality. If it is, you

FIGURE 9-3. Tissue, like large adenoids, prevents closure of the soft palate (B) against the pharyngeal wall (C) causing denasality.

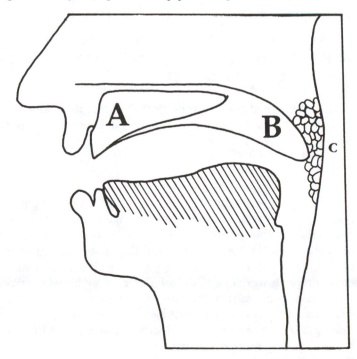

might first want to try some of the suggestions that follow for reducing the problem. If the problem persists, regardless of what you try to do, you might want to consult one of the specialists in oral-nasal-throat mechanisms listed in Chapter 16.

TESTS FOR NASALITY

There are two tests here, the first to determine if you have a problem of hypernasality and the second to determine if you have a problem of denasality. If you are uncertain which, if either, problem you have, take both tests. Neither will take long. The only equipment you need for each test is an audio cassette recorder.

Test for Hypernasality

Read aloud and record the two passages below.

EACH YEAR, EARTH SATELLITES BLAST AWAY TOWARD OUTER SPACE. THEY FLY TOWARD THE BLACK HOLE OF SPACE TO JUPITER WITH ITS CLOUDS OF ICE CRYSTALS.

BETTY WAS BOB'S BIG SISTER. SHE TOOK BOB TO THE ICE SHOW EVERY SATURDAY BY BUS. IT TOOK OVER TWO HOURS BY BUS TO REACH THE BIG CITY.

Still recording, read the passages again. But this time squeeze your nostrils closed as you begin the second sentence and continue to read aloud.

Assessing the Test Results

1. There are no nasal consonants in either of the reading passages. Consequently, on playback you should hear no nasality in your reading. If after you squeezed your nostrils closed there was no change in your voice resonance, you do not have hypernasality. Listen carefully to your recording again. If there was *no* change in the sound of your voice whether your nostrils were open or closed, you do not have hypernasality.
2. If after squeezing your nostrils closed there was a noticeable change in your resonance, or occasionally all voicing stopped, you have hypernasality. The exercises presented later in this chapter may be able to help you develop normal resonance.

Test for Denasality

Read aloud and record the two passages below.

MAN IS FINDING MANY MOONS AROUND DISTANT PLANETS. IN MANY PLANETARY SYSTEMS, MANY MOONS ARE FOUND AROUND THE NUMEROUS PLANETS.

DAN AND TOM WENT TO TOM'S GRANDMOTHER'S FARM. MANY NIGHTS ON THE FARM, THE MAN IN THE MOON SEEMED TO SHINE DOWN ON THEM.

Still recording, read the same passage again. But this time squeeze your nostrils closed as you begin the second sentence and continue reading aloud.

Assessing the Test Results

1. Both passages contain an unusual number of nasal consonants. Therefore, on the first playback, when you did not squeeze off your nostrils, the normal voice should sound quite nasal. When you squeeze off your nostrils, the normal voice will either stop completely or there will be a marked change in your nasal resonance. This would be the normal response for a voice free of denasality.

2. If you have denasality, the two recordings will sound similar. Because in denasality there is little normal nasal resonance in your voice, very little air or sound is passing through your nose when you produce m, n, and ng. Consequently, when you squeeze off your nose, if you are denasal, it will make very little difference in the way that you sound. Little or no change in voice resonance on both readings (with and without nasal pinching) shows that you are denasal, and that you might profit from the exercises for denasality presented later in this chapter.

EXERCISES FOR DEVELOPING A PROPER BALANCE OF ORAL AND NASAL RESONANCE

You now have discovered whether you have a problem of hypernasality or denasality (or no problem with nasality at all, in which case you can go on to the next chapter). The person with hypernasality will have too much nasal resonance and not enough oral resonance. The person with denasality will not resonate the nasal m, n, and ng sounds, which may impair some oral sounds as well.

The exercises that follow are designed to help you develop the right balance of oral and nasal resonance for your natural voice. They may even be useful to those of you whose problems with nasality are slight. In contrast to the examples we have used for purposes of illustration, many people are only slighty nasal or slightly denasal, and they could improve the sound of their natural voices with just a little effort.

Practice Exercises for Hypernasality

1. Lower you voice pitch a note. If you have been speaking at too high a pitch, lowering your voice to a more natural level often permits your whole vocal tract to function more efficiently. To do this, use the exercises for lowering pitch that were given in Chapter 7.
2. Reduce the loudness of your voice. A softer voice will often sound less nasal. Also, at a softer loudness level a nasal voice is less irritating to listeners. To reduce your loudness, try the exercises given in Chapter 6.
3. There should be no difference in nasal resonance when you say words that have no nasal consonants with your nostrils open or squeezed closed. Words with all oral consonants have no nasal resonance. Practice good oral resonance by saying the words listed below.

BEACH   PIG   BAKE   PORCH
PEAT   BACK   TAKE   BOOK
BITCH   PATCH   BARK   PUSH

   a. Read aloud each of the above words, one at a time, prolonging the vowel sound so the word is prolonged.
   b. Now record a second reading of the words. As you do, pinch off your nostrils now and then. If you do have hypernasality, when your nose is pinched off you will hear a marked difference in the sound of your voice.
   c. If you can hear no change in your voice when you close your nostrils, you are saying the words free of nasality. This is good. Keep up this kind of practice.
   d. If you hear any change in your voice when your nostrils are pinched closed, or if your voice is stopped, you still have too much nasal resonance and should go on to the next step.
4. Become aware of the movement of your soft palate.
   a. In front of a mirror, yawn with a wide-open mouth, breathing through your nose. Look inside your open mouth. Note

the dangling uvula hanging from your soft palate at the back of your mouth.

b. Say "AAAAAAAH," prolonging the sound. As you do, notice how your soft palate and uvula rise. At the end of the word you will see that the soft palate drops down to the open position, lowering the uvula.

c. Now say "AAAAAAANG" (rhymes with *sang*), prolonging the sound. Notice that the soft palate and the uvula stay down. This allows the sound to resonate in your nose.

d. Now say five "ah" words with your mouth wide open. Pause a second or two between each word. In the mirror you will see that the soft palate and uvula go up for each word, and drop down during the pause.

This exercise has shown you how to produce normal oral resonance. The soft palate goes up to shut off the nose from the oral cavity. When we make nasal sounds the palate drops down so that the voice can be resonated in the nose.

5. Let us take another look at the function of the soft palate, this time using a hand mirror.

a. Place the mirror directly under your nostrils. Say a prolonged "AAAAAAAH." If the sound has normal oral resonance, the mirror will not cloud from air coming from your nose.

b. Keeping the mirror in place, say a prolonged "MAAAAAAAN." As you do, you should notice the mirror cloud over from the warm, moist air coming out of your nose.

c. Say the following oral words with the mirror in place. If your voice is free of hypernasality, there will be no clouding of the mirror.

BEACH	TAKE	COURT
PITCH	DAYS	GOLD

d. Say the following nasal words with the mirror in place. Now you should see clouding of the mirror as you say each word.

MEAN	NAME	SONG
MINE	NONE	RING

6. If you said the six oral words in step c with no clouding of the mirror, see if you can make a contrast between an oral word

and a nasal word. You no longer need to use the mirror. Tape-record these pairs of words and see if you can hear a difference on playback.

TEA	KNEE	BOAT	NOTE
BET	NET	BOOK	NOOK
TAIL	NAIL	TOT	NOT
BILE	MILE	BEAR	MARE
TASK	MASK	TOYS	NOISE

When you can say these contrasting words and easily hear the difference between oral and nasal resonance on playback, you are ready to do some oral reading practice.

7. Go back to the Tests for Nasality. Record your reading of the all-oral passage. On playback, does your resonance sound normal? If you still hear some hypernasality, repeat the first six steps of these practice materials. If what you hear sounds normal to you, reinforce your progress by reading and recording the sentences below, which have no nasal consonants.

WE WISH TO SEE THE BLACK PIRATE SHIPS.
SHE ATE COTTAGE CHEESE WITH BISCUITS FOR BREAKFAST.
THE CUP OF BLACK COFFEE HIT THE SPOT.
WE DUG A HOLE FOR THE CASH BY THE GRAVEYARD.
HE WROTE THE BAD BOY A CHECK FOR FIFTY DOLLARS.
JACK TOOK JILL UP THE HILL TO LOOK AT THE VIEW.
HE TRIED TO HAVE THE COURAGE TO STOP THE BLOOD.
THEY TOOK THE SOLDIERS TO THE SAILOR'S HOSPITAL.

If your oral reading sounds free of nasality, keep practicing with any reading material that you wish. What you need at this point is continuous practice until the proper balance of oral and nasal resonance becomes second nature to you. If none of the preceding steps have helped your voice, you may need to consult some of the specialists listed in Chapter 16.

Practice Exercises for Denasality

If you found that your voice resonance was denasal on the Tests for Nasality, it is important for you to find out whether the condition is caused by physical blockage or is functional. The following screening test will enable you to determine this.

Screening Test for Denasality

Take in a bigger than normal breath. Close your mouth and let the air slowly out your nose. Now press your left nostril closed with your finger. Does the air then flow through the open right nostril? Release the left nostril and press shut the right nostril. Does the air divert through the left nostril? Do this a few times to be certain of the results.

If there is some kind of structural blockage, little air will flow through one or both nostrils. It could be caused by adenoids, swelling from allergies, or a number of other causes that need to be pursued medically (see Chapter 16). If there is structural blockage, the exercises below will not help. But, if you have found that you have good passage of air out of the nostrils yet still sound denasal, the exercises below should help you develop normal resonance.

1. Speak in a slightly higher pitch. Elevate your pitch one note, as described in Chapter 7. If the higher pitch improves your resonance, practice some oral reading using the higher pitch. Record your readings so that you can listen to your resonance critically.
2. Increase the loudness of your voice. Increasing your loudness requires greater air flow and air pressure, and this alone can help you increase your nasality. Use the exercises described in Chapter 6 for increasing your loudness.
3. Ear training is sometimes helpful for increasing nasality. For someone with a problem of denasality, *m* sounds like *b*, *n* sounds like *d*, and *ng* may sound like *g*. Ask someone with normal resonance to record the following pairs of words that denasal people often have problems with.

MAY	BAY	MAT	BAT
ME	BEE	MILK	BILK
MET	BET	MOAT	BOAT
MEAT	BEET	MORE	BORE
MY	BYE	MUST	BUST
NEED	BEAD	BING	BIG
NIP	DIP	BANG	BAG
NINE	DINE	BRING	BRIG

NO	DOUGH		RANG	RAG
NOR	DOOR		TANG	TAG

This discrimination exercise should let you hear the difference between a nasal word and an oral word when you play back the recording. Can you hear the difference? Ask the person making the recording to say just one of the words in some of the pairs. On playback, can you hear which of the words was said?

Now read and record the word pairs and the single words yourself and listen to yourself in the same critical way.

4. Try this humming exercise. Prolong an "AH" and then close your lips while you say it. The sound should then go through your nose. This is the "emmmmmmm" or humming sound.
   a. Prolong the humming *m*. Place your fingers on the bridge of your nose as you do. You should feel the nasal vibrations.
   b. Now prolong an *n* sound so that it comes out "ennnnnnn." Open your lips and place your tongue behind your upper teeth as you do. Prolong the sound as long as you can, and check the vibrations in your nose with your fingers. These vibrations represent the nasality you want to add to your voice.
   c. Now prolong an "ang" sound by saying the word "rang" and stretching it out as long as you can. Again feel your nose vibrations with your fingers.

With some practice you will soon be able to feel, even without having to check with your fingers, when the sounds you make have nasal vibrations and when they do not. This will make it easier for you to get normal nasal resonance on the words and sounds that require it.

5. If you have been successful thus far in getting some nasal sound, practice reading aloud, while recording, the two passages below that contain many nasal sounds. Make your voice extra nasal as you read, checking the vibrations in your nose with your fingers if you have to.

ON A CLEAR NIGHT, DAN AND TOM COULD SEE THE MAN IN THE MOON. ON TOM'S GRANDMOTHER'S FARM, THERE WERE MANY NIGHTS WHEN THERE WAS NO SMOKE AND SMOG. DAN AND TOM WOULD COME TO THE FARM ON MANY MOONLIT NIGHTS TO SEE THE MOON.

MAN IS FINDING MANY MOONS AROUND NUMEROUS PLAN-
ETS. IN SOME SOLAR SYSTEMS THERE ARE NUMEROUS
MOONS CIRCLING MANY OF THE DISTANT PLANETS THAT
ORBIT AROUND THE SUN.

If you have been able to increase the nasality in your voice, you now
need to spend time practicing reading and speaking with that increased
nasal resonance. Use any newspaper, magazine, or book for practice
until you feel that you have the proper nasal resonance whenever you
want it. Check your voice from time to time with your tape recorder.

Again, if your denasality has not improved, and may be related to
some kind of structural blockage, you probably should consult an otolaryngologist (ear-nose-throat doctor).

A normal, natural voice has the proper balance between nasal and
oral resonance. In the English language we need to be able to make both
kinds of sounds. To speak properly, and intelligibly, we need control
over these sounds so that they are not confused with one another. Hypernasality is a far more common problem than denasality, but denasality can be just as hard on those who have to listen to it. In most cases,
both conditions are correctable. Perhaps no voice problems are more
annoying to listeners than those related to nasality.

CHAPTER 10

Keeping Your Natural Voice Under Stress

"The stress was bad enough. What was worse was that they could hear it in my voice."

Everyone experiences stress. We all read about it and talk about it, but few of us know what it is. We also know that some of us handle it better than others. So it is not one of those things, like the weather, that "everyone talks of but nobody knows anything about."

The term *stress* was popularized a few years ago by Hans Selye in his classic book, *Stress Without Distress* (1974). After years of studying stress and stress reactions in his laboratory in Vienna, Selye concluded that "stress is the nonspecific response of the body to any demand made upon it." More simply, stress is overstimulation of the body.

Contrary to the popular view that stress comes only from negative experiences, Selye wrote that stress can come from either unpleasant or pleasant experiences. That is important to remember when it comes to voice. Elation and positive excitement can change your voice for the worse as much as anxiety. Stage fright, for example, which we deal with separately in the next chapter, might be described as both a pleasant and unpleasant experience, both exhilarating and anxiety-producing. Both emotions can have an adverse effect on voice.

All stress can change your voice, usually for the worse. About two-thirds of all voice disorders that we treat in voice clinics have no organic cause. In many of these cases, our clients are using their voices in a faulty manner, usually with too much effort, often as a reaction to stress.

It is possible, however, to maintain your natural voice even under stress. Take the case of Dorothy.

After working in an office for a number of years, Dorothy decided to try her hand in the more lucrative field of sales for the same firm. Almost immediately she began to feel the pressure of being paid strictly on commission, of not knowing how much she might make each month, not knowing if she would be able to meet her expenses or be able to budget or plan.

She became acutely aware of other aspects of her new job too. Instead of spending the day in a comfortable, air-conditioned office, she was on the road most of the time, calling on customers in all kinds of weather and, if she wanted to make money, for longer hours. The latter caused a few problems at home with her husband and son. They tried not to show it, but she knew they resented the fact that she gave them less attention than before.

Dorothy's sales record in the first few weeks on the job seemed to confirm that she would be good at selling, but the cumulative pressures at work and at home began to take their toll. She developed headaches, occasional dizzy spells, and a disposition that didn't help matters with her clients or her family.

Just as serious, the pressure also began to take a toll on her major selling tool: her voice. At times it seemed to her that it was someone else's: higher than her normal pitch, sometimes hoarse, always strained, and with occasional breaks. Toward the end of the day her voice was weak, and she had pain in her neck and throat. It started to cost her sales, a lot of them.

Someone with a less resolute character than Dorothy might have taken the easy way out and gone back to her old, salaried position. Instead, she sought help. A speech pathologist told her what she'd already guessed, that her voice problems came from stress. He also told her what she didn't know, that she could learn techniques that would help her control her voice under stress.

The results of her determination were rewarding. With the help of some exercises described later in this chapter she was able to get back her old relaxed, natural voice, and a very persuasive one it was. A stress counselor also showed her ways to reduce stress in areas where she could, and to cope with it better when she couldn't. It didn't hurt that both her company and her family saw Dorothy's commissions rise steadily each month.

But before any of us can find ways to control the voice symptoms of stress, we need to identify some of the causes of stress, what Selye called *stressors*. Let us look first at physical stressors. In most cases, we can control them to some extent, or compensate for them, at least to the point of minimizing their effects on voice.

Physical Stressors

Cold and Heat

Environments that are too warm or too cool, or too dry or too moist, clothing that is inappropriate for the temperature around us, and not drinking enough liquids are all things that can physically stress us to the point of affecting our voices.

Infection and Irritation

Fevers, rashes, itching, and inflammations of all kinds stress the body, which then struggles to maintain homeostasis (equilibrium). Discomfort or distress is reflected in how we speak, either as a direct result of the infection or irritation or because such aggravations affect our mood.

Noise and Visual Pollution

Excessive noise around us can produce strong stress reactions, as can inadequate, excessive, or irregular light, such as that caused by malfunctioning fluorescent ceiling lights (which often annoyingly buzz or hum, too). We may not be fully aware of these things, particularly if they are usual in our environment, but they can stress us enough to affect our voices.

Dietary Excesses

Eating too little, or too much, or eating things that don't agree with us can give us unpleasant or uncomfortable sensations that can be termed stressful and can affect how we speak. People who do a great deal of public speaking are aware of this. A well-known toastmaster told me once, "If I'm careful what I put into my mouth at a banquet, I don't have to worry what comes out of it later."

Recreational Excesses

Too much or too little exercise can work against physical homeostasis, creating symptoms of muscle and joint pain, stiffness, or weakness, all stresses that can show up in the voice. Excessive smoking or use of alcohol also stresses us, not only at the time we overindulge, but in the famous "morning after." The highs produced by drugs like marijuana and cocaine are followed by extreme lows, which are stress reactions.

Any of these physical stressors can result in physical or psychological symptoms that can in turn affect the voice, even if the voice isn't directly affected by them. In cases where physical stress cannot be avoided, you can, as you will see later in this chapter, do something to lessen its impact on your voice.

Situational Stressors

Certain situations in which we find ourselves produce stress reactions that may negatively affect voice. We may try to avoid some of these situations. We may try to change them to lessen the stress. But some situations we cannot change; stress comes with the territory, so to speak. In these cases we can try to learn some techniques to maintain our natural voice. The same is true for stress situations that are basically positive. We don't want to avoid these situations, or change them, but we do want to minimize any negative effect they have on our voice.

Monotony

A monotonous situation, such as a nonchallenging, repetitive job, can produce stress reactions. Even if your job basically isn't a monotonous one, most jobs have a tedious part to them. Writing this book, for example, is exciting work. Checking over the manuscript for typos, punctuation, and grammatical errors is dull. We encounter monotony in social situations too. There are dull parties and dull people we are obliged to make conversation with. These situations create stress, and stress can take its toll on our voice, often when we don't want it to. At our jobs, or in our social lives, it is usually not a good idea to let our voices betray that we are bored.

Creativity

Doing something creative, like painting, writing, or designing, can do wonders in reducing stress. If you do these things professionally, however, they can also create stress. We may develop anxiety about the quality of what we are doing or about how the work will be received. The same is true for the performing arts, but the effects of stress are more visible — and audible. The nature of creative work seems to be that it can be both stimulating and therapeutic, both anxiety-producing and enervating, and our voices may reflect it, sometimes adversely.

Depression or Sadness

Genuine depression or sadness, such as that which comes from profound loss, disappointment, or failure, needs to be expressed. But such reactions should not continue indefinitely. Certainly in daily life we do not want such emotions to always be present in our voices. We should also be aware that persistent stress reactions, such as crying, brooding, or self-imposed isolation, can become stressors themselves. In other words, we can have stressful reactions to our stressful reactions. We become sad about being sad, depressed about being depressed. And any voice problem that results can likewise be compounded.

Poverty, Racism, or Sexism

Extreme and persistent poverty or financial difficulties can color and influence all our reactions, including voice, and make matters worse. Racism also sends powerful negative stressors to those who suffer it, as does sexism, whether it originates from a man or a woman. All of these things cast a shadow over our personalities that can change the way we speak. Our responses to these situations may be realistic. Injustice, unfairness, and bad luck are never easy to take. But it is rarely to our advantage, over time, to let this show, and our voice is one of the first places it does show.

Joy or Victory

One can experience positive stress from unexpected joy, the rush of victory, or, as we discussed above, the exhilaration of creative work. But our reactions sometimes need to be controlled in order to mask our high emotional state from those around us, for instance, when we lose a contest, in negotiations, or simply to maintain the poise that is expected of those who succeed. Bad winners are as hard to bear as bad losers.

In all of the situations described, we are largely concerned with control of the voice under stress. In a moment we will show you how to gain that control. But it needs to be pointed out now that failure to control stress reactions in the voice can create further problems, and thus generate more stress. And nowhere does this seem more true than in occupational stress.

Occupational Stressors

All occupations can be stressful at one time or another. The stress can be physical, situational, or some combination of both. For some would-be blithe spirits, *any* occupation is stressful, but we will not be listening to their voices.

Some occupations, however, are inherently more stressful than others, to the point where we can only nod sympathetically when we hear someone who works in one of them say, "This job will be the death of me yet." In some occupations, like policemen, firemen, and test pilots, that can literally be true. In others, like doctors and nurses, it can be true for those they serve.

In less dramatic ways, many jobs carry heavy responsibilities for the welfare of others. The owners or chief executive officers of companies have many people's livelihoods in their hands. And, at the very least, all working people with families bear the responsibility for the welfare of their loved ones.

It is also a truism that the greater your success the greater your responsibility, whatever your line of work. The truth isn't just that "the bigger you are the harder you fall." At the headiest heights, when you fall you inevitably take some people with you.

Even those who have let go of formal responsibilities in the workplace are not relieved of stress. For many years researchers have known that retirees don't automatically start enjoying the "soft life," when they stop working. Greater pleasure from leisure and recreations is often undercut by worries about health, financial problems, and a general feeling of a lack of worth. Being retired, many senior citizens tell us, can be a full-time job, and a stressful one.

In all the above cases, voice is particularly vulnerable to stress. And in almost every job voice communication is important. A poor or inadequate voice can profoundly affect how well you perform your work. Imagine a surgeon whose orders to a nurse were as incomprehensible as, by popular belief, his scribbles on a prescription pad. Imagine a test pilot who could not tell the control tower what was wrong with his plane, a policeman or fireman who could not be understood by a fellow officer in a time of crisis. Imagine, too, a company executive who could not convey his feelings about his firm, its products, his employees, or the quality of their work, or whose voice sent signals he didn't intend or want to send.

For people in any occupation, particularly those who regularly work what have come to be called "fifteen-round days," control of the voice under stress is crucial. But it is just as crucial, and far more difficult to achieve, for those of us who face stress less frequently and, as is usually the case, unexpectedly.

Let us look now at the voice symptoms of stress and how we can learn to control them.

Voice Symptoms of Stress

Most of us are aware of the *general* symptoms of stress:

- anger
- angina
- cold hands
- confusion
- headaches
- heart disease
- heartburn
- high cholesterol
- high blood pressure
- indigestion
- loss of coordination
- ringing in the ears
- sexual problems
- sleep problems
- excessive sweating of body or hands
- tight feeling in the chest
- ulcers

Most people experience one or more of these symptoms at one time or another. They may be related to stress or they may not be. Any one of them could need the attention of your doctor. Whatever the case, if you have any of these symptoms on a regular or intermittent basis, you are also likely to display some of the symptoms of stress in your voice.

If you do, the obvious solution is to eliminate or reduce the stressors that are causing the problem. But, as we saw earlier, this is not always possible. What we must do then is learn to control stress reactions in our voices, to substitute voice control for voice symptoms of stress.

Listed alphabetically below are the 20 most common symptoms of stress in the voice. After you read them, we will show you how to overcome such symptoms to regain and retain your natural voice.

- breathy voice
- double voice (diplophonia)
- dry mouth and throat
- harshness
- high pitch
- hoarseness (dysphonia)
- lifting up of larynx
- loud voice
- low pitch
- monotone
- no voice (aphonia)
- neck or throat pain
- pitch breaks
- shortness of breath
- strained voice
- throat clearing
- tight voice
- traumatic laryngitis
- voice breaks
- weak voice

METHODS FOR KEEPING YOUR
NATURAL VOICE UNDER STRESS

Breathiness

Not all breathy voices are voices reacting to stress. The public voices of Jacqueline Kennedy-Onassis and Marilyn Monroe, for example, sounded this way all the time. But whether the cause is stress or not, a breathy voice can be changed to a natural one by the following strategies:

1. Saying fewer words per breath (see Chapter 5).
2. Raising your pitch one note (see Chapter 7).
3. Speaking with greater focus — getting your voice out of your throat (see Chapter 8).
4. Trying to speak louder (see Chapter 6).
5. Trying to speak with more precision — using a harder glottal attack (see Chapter 4).

It should be noted that a voice that has always been normal and then becomes breathy should be investigated by an ear-nose-throat doctor.

Double Voice (Diplophonia)

Occasionally people speak with two voices at once, the rather aptly named diplophonia. Often they have a low voice and a high voice blended together, which we usually perceive as hoarseness. Such a voice may occur only in moments of extreme negative stress. It can be eliminated by the following:

1. Speaking at a slightly higher pitch (see Chapter 7).
2. Using the yawn-sign to open up the vocal tract (see Chapters 10 and 11).
3. Sitting or standing tall, with the head slightly down, as if the crown of the head were suspended by a rope from the ceiling (see Chapter 4).

Dry Throat and Mouth

A typical reaction to excessive negative stress is a dry throat and mouth. If humidity levels in a room or office can be increased, this can help. Situational dryness of the throat and mouth, often related to anxiety, can be minimized by the following strategies:

1. Moving your tongue across your teeth and biting down gently on your tongue as the tongue moves around the mouth. This increases salivation.
2. Drinking 10 to 12 glasses of liquids daily. This increases your physical hydration level, and often increases the saliva in your mouth.
3. Breathing through your nose, not your mouth.
4. There are several over-the-counter sprays (Salivart, Roxane Saliva Substitute) that can keep the mouth and throat moist for several hours. They are nonsystemic solutions with no known side effects. Ask your pharmacist about them.

Harshness

This is the tense voice that is a common stress reaction for the person who "has had it." It usually occurs after exposure to prolonged, continuing stressors. The voice sounds aggressive and is difficult to listen to. The harsh voice can be replaced by the following strategies:

1. Use the yawn-sigh. Practice speaking on the sigh. There is no harshness in the sigh voice.
2. Practice keeping an open mouth while listening, reading, or watching TV, not agape, which could create a dry mouth, but with the lips slightly apart and with a relaxed jaw.
3. Dropping your pitch level one note will often make your voice sound softer.
4. Keep your head looking slightly down. Avoid extending the head upward. This helps relax the neck and throat muscles.
5. You might practice neck relaxation by rolling your head in a circle. Start with your chin down. Roll your head to the left, then up and across to the right in a circle, and down and across. Continue rolling your head seven or eight times in one direction, then reverse directions.

High Pitch

A typical stress reaction is raised pitch. If you become aware that your pitch is consistently too high, go back to Chapter 7 and follow the procedures for both finding your natural pitch and lowering your pitch level. A high speaking pitch is usually the result of excessive vocal tract tension. Lowering your pitch can be helped by the following exercises:

1. Make a conscious effort to use a lower pitch. (This is often all that you need to do.)
2. The yawn-sigh is a vocal tract relaxer and is helpful in lowering pitch.
3. Tilt your chin slightly down as you speak, and avoid extending the chin upward.
4. Make an effort to open your mouth more as you speak.

Hoarseness (Dysphonia)

Anyone who has had a normal voice and then suddenly becomes hoarse, yet doesn't have an allergy or a cold, can be displaying symptoms of a serious laryngeal disease. Anyone who is hoarse for more than 10 days should have an ear-nose-throat examination. Situational hoarseness that arises as a reaction to stress can be eliminated by the following strategies:

1. Just *trying* to speak without hoarseness will sometimes eliminate it. Often with a little effort you can listen to yourself closely and eliminate hoarseness.
2. Elevate your pitch one note.
3. Say fewer words per breath. Renew your breath by pausing when you speak (see Chapter 5).
4. Develop greater oral focus. Get your voice out of your throat (see Chapter 8).
5. At the end of a phrase or sentence, elevate your pitch.

Lifting Up the Larynx

Similar to a reaction to fear, the larynx may rise slightly as a reaction to stress. This can elevate pitch and cause the voice to become strained. If elevation of the larynx is part of a stress reaction, the following exercises might be helpful.

1. The yawn-sigh will usually lower the larynx. When we yawn, the larynx drops to a lower position. It stays in this low, normal position as we voice the sigh.
2. Tilt your head slightly down toward the chest. Open your mouth two fingers wide between your front teeth. Now practice taking in deep breaths, keeping your head down and your

mouth open. This usually relaxes the vocal tract, and the larynx remains low.
3. Speak one note lower.

Loud Voice

Often as a reaction to stress the voice may become too soft or too loud. If you find that in certain situations sometimes your voice is loud enough and sometimes it is not, you might try the following:

1. If your voice is too soft:
   a. Say fewer words per breath. Renew your breath more often.
   b. Make a conscious effort to speak louder.
   c. Elevate your speaking pitch one note.
   d. Use greater oral focus, and get your voice out of your throat.
2. If your voice is too loud:
   a. Make a conscious effort to speak softer.
   b. Lower your voice pitch one note.

Low Pitch

Some people speak at the very bottom of their pitch range as a reaction to stress. Speaking at such a low pitch usually reduces voice quality and makes your voice harder to hear and understand, particularly in noisy situations (which can cause stress to begin with). If your problem is low pitch under stress, the following exercises might be helpful.

1. Make a deliberate effort to speak a few notes above your bottom note.
2. Eliminate any throat voice focus you have. By developing good oral focus, so that your voice sounds as if it is coming off the surface of your tongue from the middle of your mouth, you will find it easier to achieve a higher pitch.

Monotone

Even people who most of the time have very spontaneous voices may develop a monotone under conditions of stress. A monotone lacks variations in both pitch and loudness. The rhythm and timing of speech sounds fixed and artificially steady. Becoming aware of a monotone is the first step for getting rid of it. Then making a conscious effort to vary pitch, loudness, and rhythm will often eliminate the monotone.

1. Practice some of the pitch inflection suggestions in Chapter 7.
2. Listen to a tape recording of your speech. Keep adding changes in inflection and volume until you don't hear the monotone anymore.

No Voice (Aphonia)

Total lack of voice can develop as a result of continued stress. This cannot be dealt with in a book such as this. Instead you should consult a speech-language pathologist or an ear-nose-throat doctor.

Pain in Neck and Throat

It is difficult to localize pain in the throat or neck. Although neck or throat pain can be solely the result of too much muscle exertion because of the way you speak, it can also be an early warning symptom of a serious medical problem. To be on the safe side, you should discuss any neck and throat pain with your doctor.

Pitch Breaks

Pitch breaks can be up or down. The voice usually breaks in the direction where it would like to be. If you are speaking too low, the voice breaks up, usually an octave higher. If you are talking too high, the voice may break downward. When pitch breaks are a reaction to stress, they can be wholly eliminated by changing your pitch level by one note. If your voice is breaking downward, lower your speaking pitch a note. For upward pitch breaks, raise your pitch a note. It should be pointed out that pitch breaks are a common phenomenon in young boys nearing the end of puberty. These pitch breaks are normal and usually disappear completely after three or four months.

Shortness of Breath

Sometimes people who usually have normal breathing become short of breath as a response to stress. They may have difficulty talking during these times, literally running out of air. If this is a problem of yours, and it is a very common one, try the following strategies.

1. Cut in half the number of words you try to say on one breath. Renew your breath more often by pausing more often.
2. Try to speak louder. This may help your breathing.
3. Speak at a slightly higher pitch.

Strained Voice

Some people react to stress by developing a strained voice. The voice becomes tight, often high-pitched and harsh, and is difficult to hear and understand. Anything that can be done to relax the vocal tract will reduce voice strain.

1. The yawn-sigh approach is the most useful technique we have for reducing voice strain.
2. Avoid looking upward. When you speak tilt your chin down slightly.
3. Practice simultaneously chewing and talking (see Chapter 11).
4. Develop a more open mouth (see Chapter 10).

Throat Clearing

Some people clear their throats excessively as a reaction to negative stressors. For many, throat clearing becomes a habit. Unfortunately, the act of clearing the throat irritates the vocal cords. The irritated cords then exude mucous. The extra mucous builds up, and the person has a need to clear out the mucous. We then, in effect, clear our throats because we already cleared our throats. Once we make a conscious effort not to clear our throats, the vocal cord irritation lessens and so does the need to clear the throat.

1. Make an effort not to clear your throat.
2. If you have a strong need to clear your throat, try to do it as silently as you can (see Chapter 4). Silent throat clearing is far gentler on the vocal cords.

Tight Voice

The methods we described for reducing voice strain also apply to the tight voice. The yawn-sigh, open mouth, and chewing approaches are usually effective in relaxing the tight voice in certain situations.

Traumatic Laryngitis

This is the temporary laryngitis (loss of voice) we get after excessive voice use, such as yelling at a ball game. Some people get laryngitis as a reaction to other kinds of stress. True laryngitis is the result of continued trauma of the vocal cords from yelling, screaming, or speaking in a noisy environment. The vocal cords become irritated, red, and swollen. The *only* treatment for traumatic laryngitis is complete voice rest. *Do not talk or whisper for 24 hours.* During this period of silence the vocal cords will usually recover completely.

Voice Breaks

Voice breaks are temporary loss of voice while speaking. For example, if someone wanted to say, "We are going to go on all the rides at Magic Mountain" with voice breaks, it would sound like: "We're going — — on all the rides at — Mountain." Voice breaks can develop as a reaction to stress. When they do, the following things can be done to stop them:

1. It is most important to say fewer words per breath.
2. Vocal tract relaxation can help:
   a. Use the yawn-sigh a bit.
   b. Keep the head tilted down and minimize looking upward.
   c. Keep your mouth slightly open and your teeth apart.
3. Speak less loudly.

Weak Voice

Sometimes continuous stress will result in a noticeable lack of voice volume. The weak voice often develops late in the reactions to stress symptoms. The voice sounds tired. It is low pitched with upward inflections at the end of phrases or sentences. The individual seems to be saying, "Will someone help me?" Help can come from practicing the following:

1. Say fewer words per breath and say them louder.
2. Get your voice focus out of your throat and put it up where it ought to be, on the surface of your tongue.
3. Elevate your voice pitch one note and inflect downward, instead of upward, at the end of sentences.

Remember, for any of these symptoms of stress in your voice, first do what you can to eliminate or reduce the stressors in your life. Once that is done, the exercises described in this chapter may help you find and maintain your natural voice in stressful situations.

CHAPTER **11**

Stage Fright and Related Fears

"Most of us are 'on stage' at one time or another — some of us frequently."

Stage fright is a term that describes a number of anxiety symptoms that many of us experience when speaking or performing in front of others. We know the physical symptoms well: excessive sweating of body or hands, cold hands, a flushed face, shaky knees, a need to go to the bathroom, confusion, upset stomach, a tight feeling in the chest, and a dry mouth.

Virtually any of the 20 voice symptoms of stress listed in the last chapter can happen with stage fright. Take a moment to review them. They will be familiar to any of you who have ever been "on-stage," making reports to fellow employees or supervisors, speaking in meetings of all kinds, or even performing on a real stage for those of us who pursue acting or singing.

Stage fright is a special kind of stress reaction, and that is why we have devoted a separate chapter to it. For one thing, the reactions that we call stage fright commonly arrive *in anticipation of* a stressful situation. As we all know, stage fright gets its name from the experiences of performers preparing to go on stage. Commonly they report that their stage fright is worse before the performance than during it. In fact, most seasoned professionals quickly lose those butterflies in the stomach once they are on stage, but then they are professionals at performing while most of us are not.

Another special thing about stage fright is that those preliminary signs of anxiety can show up no matter how many times a performer performs. Many other kinds of stress we can get used to, and our reactions will diminsh. Not always so, it seems, with stage fright. Yet we can all take heart from the fact that, after all these years, when Johnny Carson comes out for his monologue he frequently scratches the back of one hand and makes a number of other nervous gestures. And "the great communicator," former President Ronald Reagan, showed symptoms of stage fright at his press conferences by tilting his head, beginning his sentences with, "Well . . ." and having increased hoarseness. Both men freely tell us that after a lifetime of public appearances, they still experience the symptoms of stage fright.

Another characteristic of stage fright is the anxiety we feel when confronted by a challenge or opportunity. What causes the anxiety is fear of failing, of not doing well. At the same time, we know that if we do well we will be rewarded. The stage performer hopes for applause, even acclaim. Those of us who are on-stage in other kinds of situations, if we perform well, are perceived as people who know what we are talking about, who can get things done and motivate others to work well with us or for us. Here are some other situations where we can be on stage and suffer from stage fright.

Government Meetings

Many jobs today involve appearing before local, state, and federal government bodies: Your company wants to expand its plant? You may have to appear before government and citizen bodies to explain your firm's intentions, their impact on the environment, or why you need a zoning variance. Or your company may have learned of some ordinance or legislation that could adversely affect its business, and so you need to be heard by the city council, country supervisors, or state legislators — not all of these matters can be left to lawyers or professional lobbyists. As a resident of your community, a homeowner, or a parent, you may want to be heard by a planning commission, school board, community group, or even a city council or board of supervisors. Have you ever attended such meetings? Did you want to speak up on an issue of great concern to you? Did stage fright keep you quiet or make you present yourself poorly, or were you able to overcome it and speak well?

Professional Meetings

Thousands of associations and organizations have annual meetings where members present papers and participate in panel discussions. Do you volunteer to be part of these programs, or does stage fright hold you back? If you do speak, are you able to concentrate on what you are saying, or do you worry more about how you say it?

Business and Industry Meetings

Successful businesses today involve workers and management in a large number of meetings. You may be asked to give a report to your production team or sales staff, to review past performance, to set goals and motivate people for the future. There are always meetings with clients or customers where you have to explain past performance, future goals, product innovations, and your superiority to competitors. There are also meetings with organized labor, lots of them when a contract is about to expire. Even if you are running your own small business, periodically you will need to gather your employees together for an informal meeting.

The number of things that require meetings in today's business world seems endless, but they can be extremely important for you and your firm. During meetings, do you speak up? Are you able to say what you want to say? Are you relaxed, yet convincing when you speak?

Self-Help and Self-Study Groups

Many of us belong to groups like these nowadays, to help us in our careers, our social lives, or simply to broaden our interests. Did you ever notice how certain members of a group often dominate it because they speak more effectively? Do you have ideas too, or questions you think need exploring? Does something always seem to hold you back? Do you remain silent because of a little stage fright?

Other Fear Situations

You can probably think of many more situations than those listed above. Perhaps the most common situation where many of us first experience stage fright, and continue to experience it, is the job or promotion interview. There is a lot at stake at such times. And unfortunately, no matter how impressive your resume or performance record, or how sure you are that you can do this particular job better than anyone else, stage fright during the interview may cost you the opportunity, if you seem unsure of yourself, evasive or vague, or not the kind of person who can work effectively with others, or get them to work well with you.

Poise and presence are two qualities that are rated very highly in the business and professional world. By definition, stage fright deprives you of poise and presence.

CONTROLLING STAGE FRIGHT AND OTHER FEARS

In 1988 the Voice Foundation in New York City gave Helen Hayes its annual Sackler Award for having an outstanding voice. In accepting the award, Miss Hayes told the group that in the beginning of her theatrical career, between her stage fright and poor vocal technique (which can go hand-in-hand), she was convinced that she was known on the stage for her poor voice. She worked years to overcome the problem. And so, she said, to be awarded the Sackler Award was one of her "greatest honors" because it vindicated all of her early hard work.

Of course it never occurred to her not to make that effort. If she hadn't, she would not have had her brilliant stage career. That illustrates the point we made earlier about the special nature of those stress symptoms we call stage fright.

With other kinds of stress, we suggested that the first remedy to be considered was eliminating the stressor. We also said that in some cases this would be possible, and in others not. In the case of stage fright, very often, even most often, it is not desirable to eliminate the stress because what is causing it is a challenge or an opportunity.

It would seem ridiculous to us if a performer like Miss Hayes refused to go on stage simply because it was stressful. Likewise, who among us would want to turn down a job or promotion interview, or stay silent in important meetings when we had a major contribution to make, because of stage fright? These challenges and opportunities are stepping stones to a better future.

What we must do then is control the symptoms of stage fright, learn to cope with the fear itself, and to control its impact on the voice.

There are a couple of things about stage fright that make this easier than you might suppose. For one, remember that stage fright is largely an *anticipatory* fear; it afflicts us at its worst before we actually perform. This is a great advantage. Imagine if it worked the other way; that you had no fears at all before a speech, but they appeared when you stepped out in front of an audience. Because stage fright is largely an anticipatory fear, you have an opportunity to do something about the problem *before* you are actually on stage.

Another thing about that anticipatory fear is that it "gets the adrenaline flowing." If we can learn to control the *symptoms* of fear, we can used our "pumped-up" condition to give a better performance. A little bit of well-managed stage fright can overcome apathy and give extra electricity to your manner and the way you speak. Any tiredness slips away.

Let us look now at ways to manage stage fright both before and during your performance. After that we will show you how to keep your natural voice at such times.

Six Ways to Control Stage Fright and Other Fears

Remember that Your Listeners Want You to Succeed

When you listen to people give a speech, or make a report of some kind, you are hopeful that what they say will be useful to you. Your listeners feel the same way about you. They want you to succeed. They will overlook many of your flaws, like a cracking voice or a little sweat on your brow, for the message you have to give.

In fact, any of your signs of nervousness can be interpreted as flattering to your listeners, because they tell your listeners, in effect, "I am no different than you." Over my years in the classroom, I have noticed that students seem to feel more positively toward a speaker who shows some shyness than toward one who is glib and seemingly insensitive. So don't worry about showing a little nervousness.

Remember that We Hold Most Symptoms of Stage Fright Inside

Much nervousness is felt and not seen. In research projects at both the University of Denver and the University of Arizona, we looked at videotapes of ourselves in speech therapy and during supervisory conferences. Although we could not see signs of nervousness, such as change in heartbeat or warm blushing, as we watched ourselves on videotape, we relived and recalled the fears we had. Fortunately, most of these symptoms of fear could not be heard or seen by our listeners.

Look at the Audience Instead of Just Feeling You Are Being Looked At

There are two ways, one good and one bad, to stand before a group. The positive way is to *look out* and focus on the people in the audience. This helps you to forget yourself and focus instead on what you have to say. The bad way is to be aware of the audience *looking at you*. There is no surer way to encourage stage fright than too much self-focus before a group.

When I give a workshop or make a report at a meeting, I always pick out a few people who laugh or frown in reaction to what I say and do. I try to select people throughout the audience, so that my gaze moves around the room and is not limited to a seat or two. Wherever they sit, they must have reactive faces. They help me to focus out, not within.

Reading a paper is a poor way to overcome stage fright. If the reader looks up from the printed text, he or she is liable to find that much of the audience is no longer paying attention. There may indeed be something to be frightened about. One of the joys of communication is relishing the reactions of your listeners. They are what you have worked so hard to get. So look out instead of within.

Concentrate on Your Message

An old actor told a drama class, "If you want to avoid stage fright, learn your lines!" The actor was saying to be prepared. As the speaker, you should know your topic better than most of your audience. Do not organize your presentation for those few "experts" in the audience. Prepare your remarks for the majority of people there.

Prepare an outline for your presentation. Give yourself the freedom to speak from it rather than reading a text line by line. When we really know what we are talking about this is not hard, and we can enjoy our communication, which is one of the best ways to avoid stage fright.

It is the spontaneous talk or report that gives many of us problems. We stand up at a meeting to state a position, or to respond spontaneously to another speaker. If we quickly get in over our heads, the symptoms of stage fright may hit us. There is nothing more destructive to clear thinking than a rush of stage fright. Even in spontaneous situations, we need to think before we speak. A few moments of mental preparation can put your thoughts in order, and help you focus on what you say rather than how you are saying it. And your audience, too, will recognize a thoughtful pause for what it is, not as a sign of hesitancy or nervousness.

Replace Your Fear with Positive Thoughts

When Norman Vincent Peale wrote his classic *The Power of Positive Thinking*, he could just as well have titled the book, The Power of Negative Thinking. Negative thinking is as self-destructive as positive thinking can be self-fulfilling.

The 1990 Directory of the Natonal Speakers Association shows that most of its members present lectures and workshops on self-confidence as the first step for increasing self-fulfillment, creativity, and productivity.

Positive thinking is also an important step for overcoming stage fright. Many of our stage fright fears are over-reactions to previous situations in which we experienced symptoms of fear. You may have spoken up at a neighborhood association meeting and were unsure of yourself: Your face became flushed, your voice became tense, and you felt shaky in the knees. Since that experience, whenever you are in a group situation you fear that these symptoms will come back when you speak. That is the power of negative thinking. We generalize from an earlier unpleasant situation to a present situation.

But each speaking situation is a separate, unique opportunity. You may be speaking about different things. Your audience is different. And, most of all, *you* are different, because you are aware of that past experience and can learn from it.

A big part of positive thinking is nothing more than having the confidence that you won't repeat your past mistakes. Learning the techniques to do that allows you to change negative thinking into positive thinking.

Replace Your Fears with Relaxation Techniques

Although stage fright and other fears appear to be universal conditions, keeping them in check seems to be a common characteristic of successful people. How many people have we known who have great speaking voices in private but are almost struck dumb when they have to speak to a group? This is similar to a man who can play the piano like Van Cliburn, but only if no one is listening, or a woman who plays tennis like Chris Evert on the back courts, but can never play well in a tournament.

The big difference between the amateur performer and the pro is that the professional has learned to stay relaxed. Performance success may be at least as much a matter of "keeping your cool" under pressure as it is a matter of talent.

Here are four relaxation techniques that have proved helpful in the battle to diminish stage fright.

1. The Relaxer. Say, for example, you find yourself in a tense situation where you have to call someone on the phone with a very negative message. Before you make the call, sit in a chair with your arms hanging limp or in your lap. Drop your chin a little toward your chest with your mouth slightly open. Now close your eyes. Take in bigger, relaxed breaths, taking them in slowly and letting them out slowly. Feel the openness of your airway. Picture in your mind that your mouth is slightly open, your tongue down, and your throat wide open. Don't think of anything else. Think only of your open mouth and throat. Keep your mouth open until your jaw and face seem somewhat heavy, a normal feeling when you relax your mouth, jaw, and throat. Now when you make that tough phone call you will find your stage fright symptoms have diminished.

2. The Head Roll. Keep your body in the same position you used with The Relaxer. With your mouth slightly open, roll your head slowly from side to side. Feel the heaviness of this movement.

Now practice rolling your head in a circular, clockwise pattern. From the chin-down position, with your mouth still open, roll your head to the left and then up so that you are looking at the ceiling. Continue across to the right and down and then across again. After eight clockwise rolls, reverse direction and roll your head counterclockwise. The Head Roll is an excellent way to relax the head and neck, which can tense up when you are anxious.

3. The Invisible Yawn-Sigh. This is an old professional's technique. Unlike the two previous exercises, which would be quite visible, the Invisible Yawn-Sigh can be done on the platform. It is simple to do once you practice it a few times. Keep your mouth closed and yawn (an exaggerated inspiration of air). Now let the air out with a closed-mouth sigh (the air exits through your nose). When you yawn-sigh like this it dilates and relaxes your throat.

Experienced speakers and performers often use the Invisible Yawn-Sigh as they are being introduced on the platform or stage. Even if they are experiencing stage fright, when they speak after this exercise, their voice sounds perfectly relaxed.

4. Progressive Relaxation. One of the most effective relaxation techniques ever introduced was Jacobson's Progressive Relaxation. The technique begins by concentrating on a particular part of the body, such as the fingers or toes. Once you have isolated such a body part, say the toes, follow these steps:

a. Lie on your back with your arms and legs extended. Close your eyes and concentrate on your toes for a few moments.
b. Now curl your toes as hard as possible. Keep them contracted like this for 30 seconds. Then slowly relax them.
c. Feel the sharp contrast between the tightness you experienced when the toes were contracted with the heaviness you feel when they are relaxed. Concentrate on this heavy feeling of relaxation.

At this point you might then go on to the foot, the ankle, your hands. Some of you may have heard of these exercises as an aid in getting to sleep. They work. They also work well to get you in a physically and mentally relaxed state of mind before any situation that might cause stage fright.

Five Ways to Keep Your Natural Voice in Fear Situations

Although stage fright symptoms can be minimized by using the techniques just described, it is unlikely that any of us can completely eliminate them. Remember that many veteran performers, such as Johnny Carson and former President Ronald Reagan, report that they still experience stage fright even after all their years of speaking before the public.

Remember too what we said earlier in this chapter: The stress that provokes these symptoms can be an asset because it can give our performances that little extra bit of electricity. That is only effective, however, when we are in control of the stage fright symptoms, and have not let them control us. Nowhere is that more important than with the voice.

Voice can, to use the old expression, "betray" your feelings of nervousness and anxiety. No matter how well your manner, expression, posture, and gestures conceal your anxiety, your voice can reveal the real state you are in. Virtually none of the 20 symptoms of stress listed in the previous chapter are an asset when speaking. In fact, they all can have a very negative impact on your listeners.

Fortunately, there are a few techniques that will help you find and keep your natural voice despite feelings of fear. Some of the techniques you can only use before you go on stage — but that is when the symptoms of stage fright are often most acute. Others you can use during your performance, or just prior to speaking. Either way, by using one or several of the five techniques listed below, your voice can sound natural and relaxed.

Develop an Open Mouth and Keep Your Teeth Apart

One of the bad things some people do when they have stage fright is to bite down hard on their molars and close their mouths. Many people even attempt to go on speaking through clenched teeth. The result is a voice that sounds strained and speech that is hard to understand. Or the frightened person sometimes bites down hard and grinds his molars together (known as *bruxism*). This also contributes to overall vocal tract tension, unintelligibility — and a very uncomfortable reaction from the audience.

When you experience stage fright, make a deliberate effort to keep your mouth slightly open. Keep your back molars slightly apart. Keep your lips slightly apart. Keep this slight opening between teeth and lips, particularly when you are not talking. It will give you a relaxed feeling that will offset some of your tension.

The Chewing Method

This is another method that will help overcome the closed-mouth and clenched-teeth symptoms. It is particularly helpful for those who find this a persistent and severe problem. Look at yourself in a mirror as you count to 20. Do you open your mouth and move your lips and jaw as you speak? You should. The closed tight mouth, which can make you look like a ventriloquist, requires a lot of muscular effort, and results in a voice that is unpleasantly tense and hard to understand.

If this is a problem for you, see if the steps of the chewing method will help you.

1. Stand in front of a mirror and pretend that you are chewing three crackers at one time with an open mouth. Move your tongue around as if you were actually chewing. This exaggerated chewing (without food in your mouth) may not be attractive, but it is the first step in learning this technique. Your face will look a bit distorted, your jaw will move from side to side, and your mouth will be opened wider than usual. But this is only temporary.

2. Now add light voice, like a hum, to your exaggerated chewing. This will produce a monotonous "yum yum" sound. Do this briefly until you get the feeling of chewing simultaneously with voice. Now keep the chewing going, but instead of just humming say these two nonsense words: AHLAMETERAH and WANDAPANDA. Say them in a prolonged, chanting style, and chew them as you say them. Practice this until you feel relaxed doing it.

3. Now practice counting while you chew in the exaggerated manner. Slowly count: 1-2-3-4-5. This speaking while chewing (something our mothers told us not to do) is the start of developing normal mouth movements for speech.

4. Now practice reading a sentence or two while you chew.

5. Practice some spontaneous conversaton as you chew. Watch yourself in a mirror. If you are comfortable with the exercise now, start to cut down the exaggerated mouth movements until the movements look normal. If you are concerned with what normal is, pay attention to what actors, actresses, and announcers do on television. What are their mouths doing as they speak?

6. In voice therapy, I usually end our practice chewing-speaking by telling my client, "From this point on *think chewing* when you speak." Just thinking about it will help you remember the feeling. We then combine the chewing method with the open mouth method we discussed first.

Keep Your Natural Pitch

There is a natural tendency for pitch to rise during anxious moments. In a fear situation, the larynx may rise in the neck and the laryngeal muscles may tighten. This causes elevation of pitch. Not all people with stage fright experience this, but if you do the following steps should help.

Remember that in Chapter 7 we found that your natural pitch was usually three or four notes above the lowest note you could produce. If you find that your pitch rises during moments of stage fright, make a deliberate effort to bring it down to its natural level by following some of the pitch-lowering exercises in Chapter 7. In addition, the following tips might help you.

1. Keep your chin down and tilt your head toward your chest. It is easier to find a lower pitch with this head position.

2. Practice saying "uhm huh." Prolong the "huh" so it sounds like an "aaaaaaaaah." Now sweep it down to near your lowest pitch. You should be able to go up a note or two from this level and be able to use that level in fear situations.

Renew Your Breath More Often

When we experience stage fright or other fears, our breathing sometimes becomes more irregular. If you feel that your breathing changes when you are fearful (many people do not experience this), there are a number of things you can do to correct it. Some of them you can do just before, others even during, those times of stress.

1. Take a few deliberate long breaths. For example, as you are being introduced to speak, sit with your head slightly down and take in a long breath. Now let the air out slowly. Repeat several long breaths, in and out. It will give you much better control of your breathing.

2. Many people experience shortness of breath from stage fright, because they don't take in enough air with a breath or because they try to say too many words on each breath. The best way to renew your breath while speaking is simply to pause. During the pause, your breath will renew itself with no special effort. If you are experiencing stage fright, cut down the number of words you say on a breath. Pause. Then go on speaking. Pause again and go on speaking.

Use the Yawn-Sigh

Stage fright can often close off your throat and make your voice sound tense and bottled up. As discussed earlier, the yawn-sign is an excellent method for opening and relaxing the vocal tract. During the yawn-sigh the pharynx is maximally dilated. No matter how tight and closed off your throat may feel, if you yawn it will open up.

The procedures for the yawn-sigh are simple.

1. *Yawn.* Inhale with an open mouth. Really yawn, as you do when you are tired.

2. *Sigh.* Let the air out with a prolonged breath sigh, tongue down, mouth open, throat open. There should be a light voice on the sigh.

3. *Extend the light-voiced sigh.* As you sigh, let your regular voice come out. This should be your natural voice. After the sigh your voice should sound opened, relaxed, and somewhat back in focus.

If you feel throat tightness build up as part of stage fright, use the yawn-sign. This is a technique that you can use to relax your throat before you go on stage but it can also be used just before speaking, or even during a pause when speaking, as we described a few pages back in The Invisible Yawn-Sigh. Either method will give you an open, back voice that is a much better voice than the high, tense voice sometimes heard during stage fright.

CHAPTER **12**

Telephones and Microphones and Your Natural Voice

"You can't expect the equipment to do all the work."

With computers the basic wisdom, "garbage in, garbage out," means that the information you get from them will be no better than what you feed in. The same principle applies to telephones, microphones, and other electronic means for transmitting the human voice. These devices will not make our voices sound good, or even intelligible, if we don't give them good voice to begin with. They are, after all, only mediums of transmission. The prime instrument of communication is still your own voice.

At the same time, however, no matter how well you have learned to develop a good voice, all of that effort can be lost if you have not learned how to use such transmitting devices effectively. And many of us have not. Although we spend a good part of our waking hours on the telephone, and some of us, at least from time to time, find ourselves standing before a microphone, it is a rare person who has ever had any instruction on how to use such devices. The purpose of this chapter is to show you how.

THE TELEPHONE

Some of the most important messages we communicate are delivered by telephone. A lot of us do the bulk of our business on the phone, making decisions that involve large sums of money. In fact, it is not unusual for business relationships to be initiated and sustained solely by telephone. A retailer friend of mine once dealt with a supplier for seven years without meeting him in person until one day, on a whim, he suggested lunch. (The lunch lasted hours and the two men became close friends.)

People fall in, and out, of love because of telephone conversations. Friendships are kept alive, or broken, over the phone. People in trouble or in need depend on the telephone for comfort, reassurance, and help. In a highly mobile society such as ours the telephone is often the only thing that keeps family feelings alive between infrequent get-togethers.

How well we do at such communication varies greatly from individual to individual. Some people are "good on the phone," others are not. Some people like talking on the phone; others, even over a lifetime, dislike it and it shows in their voices. Some people feel uncomfortably "onstage" on the telephone while others use it casually and easily.

The reasons for these differences stem from two facts that are more obvious than they are appreciated. The first is that the telephone is only a voice transmitter, not a voice enhancer. If you habitually use a poor voice, and do nothing to improve it, you will have a poor voice on the telephone. Almost the only people whose speaking voices can be improved by the telephone are those who normally speak too softly.

Secondly, the only way the telephone transmits our communication is by the sound of our voice. Yet, we have all known people who are just as animated in gestures and body language in phone conversations as they are in personal conversations. That is all very well if those feelings register in their voices too. But often they do not. Such people are always surprised or upset when their phone messages are misunderstood, when the other person doesn't react to their gestures or expressions, or perhaps doesn't respond to their personality at all. The result, over time, can be a telephone voice that from the first words conveys frustration, resentment, and even anger.

Other phone users are comfortable with the fact that such visual clues to their personalities are unseen. They even count on it, and often develop a special "telephone voice" that "sells" them. Let's face it, on the telephone no one can tell if we are fat or thin, ugly or attractive, or whether we look sincere and honest or hypocritical and shifty as we speak. If we are good with our voices, we can project in sound alone the image of ourselves that we want.

While it might seem that a person who has cultivated a beguiling telephone voice has an advantage, often this is not the case. Many a man or woman has made a business or social date with one of those great sounding telephone voices only to be badly let down in person. And the experience is no more pleasant for the person who sees that let-down expression than it is for the person who is let down.

Although one voice might be heard as "good" and another as "bad," in fact, it is best not to develop a distinctive telephone voice and personality, but as in most situations in life, to speak with our natural voice. A few simple techniques can help you to present yourself as you really are, effectively convey what you mean and feel, and put you as much at ease on the telephone as you are in personal conversation.

Let us approach these techniques by examining the most common problems people encounter in using the telephone.

Voice Identity on the Telephone

People who are apprehensive or uncomfortable using a telephone frequently are convinced that the person they have called will not know who they are, even if that person knows them fairly well. Other people make phone calls with utter confidence that they will be instantly identified.

We have all had calls from both types. The first person usually gives his first name right away and often, after an uncertain pause, his last name and other identification too: "Hello. This is Randy. Randy Brown. Randy Brown from Mason Industries." If the person getting the call already knows the caller reasonably well, such an opening sounds tentative and unsure.

The second kind of caller usually doesn't give his name or, if he does, gives only a first name: "Hi. This is George. Where is the shipment you invoiced us for last Thursday?" This approach can also have a negative result, particularly if the person calling is not that well known, or if the person receiving the call deals with large numbers of people on the phone, many of whom might be named George.

The point is that identification of the caller is of major importance in telephone communication. In fact — those who are apprehensive or uncomfortable on the phone take note — the best thing you have going for you when you phone is that it is *you* making the call. The person answering recognizes who you are, who you represent, and what your business is likely to be. This quick orientation makes it possible for the conversation to go smoothly. But even when you give your name at the beginning, as you should, it is important that you continue to sound like yourself. You will also need to avoid some of the following problems.

Loudness and the Telephone

The two most common difficulties in telephone conversations are speaking too softly and speaking too loudly. While the telephone is an amplifier, and many soft-spoken people get a needed amplification boost, others make that amplification impossible by holding the transmitter too far away from their mouths, or turning their faces away from the instrument.

This is often just a careless habit. We have all seen the person who lets the transmitter part of the phone drop until it is closer to the Adam's apple than the mouth, or the person who turns his or her head to stare out the window or up at the ceiling. For the person on the other end of the line, the effect is the same as if the speaker had moved away from the phone.

On the other hand, the telephone's amplifying power can be a disadvantage for the person who speaks too loudly, or holds the transmitter too close to the mouth. The result is voice distortion. Not only does this make it difficult to identify the caller, but the person called can be as irritated by a loud, distorted voice as by a voice that is too soft to hear.

People with these kinds of problems using the telephone should remember that the instrument is designed for the adult-sized head. When the receiver is at your ear, the transmitter end of the phone extends down below your mouth, where it should be.

For most people, the best phone position seems to be what we see in Figure 12-1. The transmitter end of the phone is kept about 1 to 2 inches away from the mouth and slightly below it, by the chin. This position will give the amplification needed by soft-spoken people, but prevent distortion from all but the loudest talkers.

The best loudness level on the telephone is a light voice. Remember back in Chapter 6 when we talked about the Level 2 voice, a voice loud enough to be heard but not so loud that it would awaken someone sleeping nearby? This is the best telephone loudness level. The Level 3, conversational voice, is often too loud.

Getting the right loudness level on the telephone is relatively simple — the instrument is designed to help you. That it is a problem at all is, like other problems with the telephone speaking voice, probably due to the fact that we almost never hear our own voices on the telephone. What we hear is our normal voice, not the transmitted voice, and the latter is different.

The telephone will not carry any high frequencies beyond 3000 Hz. (A good stereo system will reproduce over 20,000 Hz.) Some of the lower tones of the adult voice are also filtered away. In addition, especially on some long distance calls, there can be static or other interference on the line. There can also be a great variation in the quality of voice reproduction depending on what telephone you use. In short, what you hear as you speak on the phone is not the voice the person you called hears. And that includes your level of loudness.

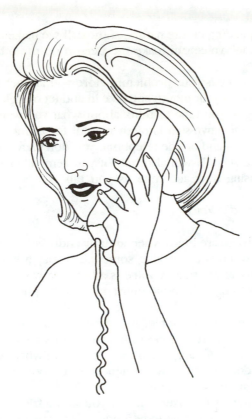

FIGURE 12-1. A good way to hold the telephone.

Those of you with telephone answering machines can test your voice loudness by dialing your machine and leaving a message. How does it sound compared to other messages you receive? If you don't have an answering machine, ask a friend or family member to rate your loudness.

After such tests, all you really need to do is stay aware of the position of the transmitter relative to your mouth, use a Level 2 voice volume, and maintain your natural pitch a couple of notes above the lowest note you can produce.

The Tense Voice

This is a common problem for people who dislike talking on the telephone and for people who are frustrated because the phone doesn't carry visual as well as sound images. But any of us can sound tense on the telephone, depending on the nature of the call we make or receive, and a tense telephone voice can make the person on the other end of the line tense.

If a tense voice is your problem, before you answer the telephone or make a call open your mouth and take in and let out a few big breaths. This will also give you time to think about what you want to say. Then our old friend the yawn-sigh is often helpful for maintaining a relaxed telephone voice — and on the telephone you don't have to worry about the yawn being seen. It will also help if you remember to renew your breath by pausing now and then as you talk.

The Unfriendly Voice

Although there are times when an unfriendly voice on the phone is called for (as when you're asking someone to pay a bill for the umpteenth time), usually a friendly voice is a better way to get things done. But some of us frequently sound unfriendly on the phone, even without meaning to.

This can be just a matter of not paying attention to what we are doing. After all, most telephone calls arrive unexpectedly. We may be concentrating on something or someone else, and when we pick up the telephone we don't make an adjustment in our mood or voice, or are a little irritated at the interruption.

To gain some control over whether you sound friendly or unfriendly on the phone, try this simple experiment. Use your telephone answering machine, or ask a friend or relative to help. When you speak on the phone deliberately smile as you speak. Then deliberately frown — it is virtually impossible to do both at the same time. Now listen to the recording of your voice, or ask a friend or relative if those changes in expression were reflected in your voice. Most of the time the difference between a smiling and a frowning voice is obvious.

If it is to your advantage to sound friendly on the telephone, speaking with a smile can help. You can prepare for it by thinking about something pleasant. It also helps to remember that, just as it is important to you to be recognized on the telephone, recognition is important to others too. When you visualize the person on the other end of the line, a more personal feeling will be heard in your voice.

The Unconcerned Voice

This might be termed passive unfriendliness. The person using this voice sounds cool or cold, impersonal. You may have noticed that even some of the people you know well speak this way on the telephone.

They sound as if they are talking to a stranger, and you want to say, "Wait a minute. This is *me*."

Such a voice often belongs to a person who feels that a conversation with a person they can't see, and who can't see them, isn't a real conversation at all. But it is also common among people who are overworked, harassed, or who have to spend a great deal of time on the telephone. What comes through is that they are just making, or receiving,"another call," rather than talking to an individual.

The best corrective action, particularly when you have been having a hectic day, is to take a moment before you make a call or answer the telephone to visualize the person you are going to speak with, and accommodate your voice for that person. You can reinforce this personalization by using the other person's name with some frequency in the conversation, instead of just delivering your message. This is also the time for you to deliberately improve your mood before a call, and use the smile when you are talking. A friendly voice is never an unconcerned voice.

The Scared Voice

It might seem strange in this technological age, but there are some people who are frightened of using the telephone. They are nervous when it rings. They make calls reluctantly. Before they dial they may rehearse what they plan to say or clear their throats. When they speak they sometimes seem to be "trying on" different voices, looking for the right one to use. In short, the frightened person sounds nervous, uncertain, and uncomfortable. If they are usually frightened of people, then the problem is not in the phone. But if they generally relate well to people but have a problem doing so on the telephone, then it has become the primary obstacle to communication.

Here are a few ways to desensitize such a "phone phobia." First, remember that the telephone is just a plastic, electronic instrument designed to convey your voice messages. Its sole purpose is to make communication easier for you, not harder.

Second, practice speaking on the telephone by unplugging it but pretending you are talking on a "live" phone. Practice speaking or reading aloud on the disconnected instrument until you feel more comfortable doing it.

Then, third, reconnect the telephone and call either your answering machine or a friend, relative, or family member. Try to maintain the ease that you achieved when you spoke into the disconnected phone.

As in some of the previous problems we have discussed, another way to overcome "phone phobia" is to visualize the person you are calling, or who has called, and to personalize the conversation by using the person's name. Often this will cause the other person to use your name more frequently, which will put you more at ease too.

Finally, for those of you with a serious case of "phone phobia," review Chapter 11, Stage Fright and Related Fears. The same relaxation techniques that work before a live audience will help you with the electronic device called a telephone.

A last tip. Oddly enough, people who have a fear of the telephone are often the ones who snatch it up on the first ring or grab it impulsively when they decide to call someone. Perhaps they are just trying to get it over with. But if they want to get rid of the fear in their voices, the best thing they can do is take a moment before answering or making a call to reflect on the techniques we have described above.

Being Understood on the Telephone

Any of the problems we have just talked about can make it difficult for you to be understood on the phone. That is obviously the case when you speak too loudly or too softly. But if your telephone voice is tense, unfriendly, impersonal, or scared, you may have problems being understood too. Such qualities can be so distracting to the person on the other end of the line that he or she may miss your message. When someone asks you to repeat something you have said, it may be because they were thinking of something else when you spoke. That something else could well be the way you were speaking.

Moreover, if the person you are speaking with thinks he knows you, but your voice sounds "different," that can also be distracting. Most people who know your voice, or think they are expected to, are reluctant to ask bluntly, "Who is this?" As a result, while you are delivering your message they may be trying to identify your voice.

As a general rule, even with people you know well, it is best to open your end of the conversation by mentioning your name. Those who know you well won't mind, and those who don't will appreciate it.

Telephone Accessories

There are a number of attachments available that are designed to make your telephone more convenient to use. Some of them may help you overcome some of the problems we discussed above; others bring with them new problems or aggravate existing ones.

The *telephone answering machine* irritates many people. We dial a number expecting to talk to a person but what we get is a recorded, and sometimes cute and lengthy message, instructions on when to speak, and in the case of some machines, even how long a message we can leave.

Like the telephone itself, these devices are designed to aid communication. They can be a blessing for many small businesses or professional offices, or for any of us who are not always available to take a call.

The recorded message is only telling us that the person we have called wants to hear from us. If you really want to talk to that person, or business, it behooves you to speak as well to the machine as you would to the person. As much can be riding on the message you leave on tape as if you had delivered it in person. Any irritation with the machine can be interpreted as irritation with the other party.

Hearing and speech amplification devices are available on many phones. The former are very useful if the person on the other end of the line speaks too loudly or softly, or if you are hard of hearing. The latter can help you if you are the one with a problem of speaking too softly.

The *speaker phone* is a feature available for many of today's telephones. It is useful for people who want to do something with their hands, such as take notes or type, while taking or making a call. It is also useful when you want others to hear what is said on an incoming call.

A good number of people, however, use this feature for casual convenience. They want to pour themselves another cup of coffee, look out the window, or just stroll around. The results can be dismaying. Most speaker phones make the voice sound as if it were coming out of a bank vault or the bottom of a well, and make it sound more impersonal as well. Moving around while using a speaker phone can also markedly affect intelligibility.

A speaker phone does give you mobility, but not unlimited mobility, and not without consequences for voice quality. If you like to use a speaker phone, you should test the one you have by calling your answering machine, or a friend or relative, and testing how your voice sounds on it at various distances from the transmitter.

Cordless and cellular phones give you much more geographical mobility than a speaker phone since they are designed to work hundreds of feet from the home unit, or over a distance of miles in the case of the cellulars. On the better sets your voice will also be as clear as it is on a regular telephone. But there are many cheaper sets on the market that seriously compromise the quality of your voice, whatever your distance from the home unit. In the case of cellular phones there can be a lot of extraneous noise on a call too, from traffic if you are in a car or from other sources if you are calling from a boat. Moreover, many of the cordless sets are vulnerable to interference from radio transmitters and other nearby callers using cordless phones. People using cellular phones while driving can find themselves suddenly in an area where transmission or reception vanishes.

With any telephone accessory, the rule is that you should test the equipment thoroughly before you commit to buying it. If your telephone calls are important to you, you don't want to add anything to your phone equipment that makes your voice sound worse or that could be aggravating to the person on the other end of the line.

The Microphone

Mike fright is a term that originated in the early days of radio, and refers to the same kinds of symptoms that we read about as stage fright. For many people, the mere sight of a microphone is enough to make them panic.

But a microphone used well can enhance one's voice and greatly facilitate communication between a speaker and an audience. Indeed, before sizable groups, and in large rooms, a microphone is necessary to communicate at all.

A good public address (PA) system, consisting of microphone, amplifier, and speakers, has far greater audio fidelity than a telephone. It can pick up all the high and low pitches of your voice, amplify its resonance, and even compensate to some extent for lack of voice focus. Some people with ineffective, or unremarkable, voices in person can sound wonderful over a PA system.

But only if they know how to use it properly. Most of us have had little or no experience using a microphone, and used poorly it can make a shambles out of what you are trying to say.

There are several types of microphones in use today. The most common type is mounted on a floor stand, with a cord running to the amplifier. Often it can be detached from the stand so the speaker is free to move around the stage or platform — if he remembers to keep his feet from getting tangled up in the cord. Whether it remains on the stand or is held in the hand, the person speaking must be constantly aware of the distance between his or her mouth and the microphone. With a sensitive microphone, even small variations in that distance can make a large difference in sound.

Another common type of microphone sits on a short stand on a lectern or is attached to the lectern. It leaves both hands free for gestures, and the mouth-to-microphone distance is relatively, but not absolutely, constant.

The cordless microphone is usually of the lavaliere (hung around the neck) or clip-on (clipped on your clothing) type. It gives the speaker maximum freedom of movement and hand gestures, with no worry about getting the feet tangled in the cord. It also has the advantage of remaining a fixed distance from your mouth and prevents unwanted variations in volume.

Different speakers prefer different styles of microphones — but rarely, for most of the readers of this book, will you have any choice of equipment. Many people, including a lot of singers, are uncomfortable without the mike as a prop in their hands. Others want the freedom a lavaliere or clip-on gives to indulge in the full range of hand and arm gestures. And some prefer the lectern mike which gives them the option of using some gestures.

The most important thing is to understand the equipment you are given to work with so that you can use it to your best advantage. We will show you how to do this. As you will see, you need to concern yourself not just with the microphone itself, but with the amplifier and loudspeakers.

Tips for Using a Microphone

Maintain good eye contact. Once you have made yourself familiar with the public address equipment, you can and should forget about it. The impression you want to convey to your audience is that you are speaking to them, not a microphone, that your audience is hearing *you* speak, not your voice coming out of the loudspeakers. So always look beyond the microphone at your audience. As far as you and they are concerned, it is not there.

Make sure the amplifier settings are right for you. The typical amplifier has controls for setting volume (also called gain) and bass and treble. You want to get these right for your voice before the audience arrives. A little more bass will give you a deeper, more resonant sound if you need it. More treble will help your voice carry better. Most of our consonants are high frequency sounds, so setting the treble higher will emphasize them and make you easier to understand.

Once you have established the right bass and treble for your voice, find the right volume setting. Because you are testing in an empty room your voice could reverberate and sound louder than it will when the absorbed. It is a good idea to have a cooperative person, whom you can signal, stand next to the amplifier to raise or lower the volume once you begin to speak.
you begin to speak.

Watch the distance between your mouth and the microphone. This is important for those using a microphone on a floor stand or a hand-held mike. But speakers facing a microphone on a lectern need to be aware of it too, because head and upper body movements alone can change the distance from the mouth to the microphone by almost a foot.

It is best to keep the microphone at chin rather than mouth level. This will prevent that occasional explosive sound that occurs if you get a little too close, and also keeps the audience from hearing you take in a breath.

There is no one distance from the microphone that is best for everyone or every situation. Our voices vary a great deal from one another — and so do amplifiers and microphones. People who work with microphones a lot have found that a distance of 6 to 12 inches works well most of the time. If at that distance your voice is too soft or too loud, it is better to change the gain on the amplifier rather than try to change the volume of your voice. Standing too close to the microphone can produce amplification squeals and voice distortion. Standing too far away can make it difficult for your listeners to hear you. Pick a comfortable mike-to-mouth distance and stick to it.

Watch for amplification/loudspeaker squeal. Usually your audience enters the room where you are to speak in a receptive mood. They are there because they want to hear what you have to say. But you can forfeit all that good will quickly if the first thing they hear is a squeal or squawk from the loudspeaker. You are the one standing at the microphone so in their minds it is somehow your fault.

In fact it is. You should have tested the equipment before the audience got there.

Loudspeaker squeal is often caused by the way loudspeakers are positioned in relation to the microphone, if the speakers are on the stage. Repositioning the microphone a little forward or farther away from the speakers will usually correct such a problem. You can also get squeal if the mike is not positioned correctly in relation to the amplifier, and solve the problem the same way.

Other causes of speaker squeal are loose connections between the microphone, amplifier, and speakers, which can also cause speaker crackle, excessive volume or treble settings, or just speaking with your mouth too close to the microphone.

Whatever the cause, the problem should be found and fixed before the audience arrives. All but the most experienced public speakers have enough worries in front of an audience without putting themselves at an additional disadvantage because they have not checked out the equipment beforehand.

If you are in a position where you cannot do that, say at a dinner banquet you have gone to after work, and at which you are expected to speak, listen carefully to the qualities of the PA system when the first speaker talks. If something is wrong, make sure someone fixes it, or fix it yourself.

Control the emotions in your microphone voice. In our chapters on stress and stage fright we gave suggestions for controlling the symptoms of fear and stress in your voice. These are particularly important when you talk on a microphone since the device can markedly amplify emotion in your voice. A tremor of apprehension or a hint of strain that might go unnoticed in ordinary conversation can be reproduced with excruciating fidelity over a good PA system. The system's amplification can also be a problem since many of us in situations of stress speak much louder than normal. Many a nervous speaker has startled an audience out of their seats by his first booming words. Changes in pitch are also common symptoms of stage fright and stress that can be exaggerated by a PA system.

If you are one of those people who get "mike fright," or if you are simply inexperienced in using a PA system, it would be a good idea to have the suggestions in Chapters 10 and 11 firmly in mind before you find yourself with a microphone between you and your audience.

Other Electronic Voice Aids

There are a number of electronic devices designed to help people with speaking and hearing disabilities, such as body amplifiers, artificial larynges, and hearing aids. For people who need them, they are blessings, but since both written and personal instructions come with their purchase, we do not need to deal with them here. However, two other electronic communication devices that have come into widespread use in recent years deserve some attention.

Citizen band (CB) radios have achieved considerable popularity for use in boats, motor homes, and recreational vehicles of all kinds, as well as in ordinary cars. The typical CB unit can transmit your voice about five miles.

The biggest voice problem with CB units (apart from the fact that many people speaking on them try to sound like truckers among whom they first became popular) is that callers talk too loudly on them. It is almost as if they feel they need to speak more loudly to span the distance between their unit and the receiving unit.

Keeping your voice at a soft Level 2 voice is generally the best voice for a CB radio, but remember that background noise from other traffic, or keeping your window open, can affect this. Remember, too, the suggestions we made about proper postioning of a microphone in relation to the mouth.

FM walkie-talkies permit voice communication between sender and receiver in a limited range, usually within a quarter of a mile or less. Since the instruments are now much smaller than they used to be, hunters and hikers often use them recreationally. In fact, recently an earpiece walkie-talkie has been developed that is a sender as well as a receiver — the microphone picks up voice vibrations from your jawbone.

The best voice for this device is also a light conversational voice, the Level 2 voice. But depending on background noise (wind is a factor outdoors), and how close you are to the limit of the range of your equipment, you may need to use a louder voice in order to be heard.

The basic thing to remember about all electronic voice equipment is that, although such devices are designed to facilitate communication, they cannot do this most effectively without some thought and effort on our part. If voice communication on them is important to us, we need to learn to use them well.

These instruments do change the way we sound and how we present ourselves to others. In the case of the telephone, for example, we are heard but not seen. In the case of the microphone, in various ways it can come between us and our listeners with a consequent loss of rapport.

We first need to understand both what the equipment is designed to do for us and how it works, what it will do and what it cannot do. We need to control it, not let it control us.

Second, we need to gain control over our voices when using such devices. Because they change the way we sound, they present challenges to the way we use our voices, challenges that are different from those we encounter in usual face-to-face communication.

None of this is difficult if you follow some of the suggestions in this chapter. And the rewards are great — and important. All of us need to use the telephone frequently in our work and social lives. And those of us with advancing careers will encounter more and more situations in which we need to use a microphone.

CHAPTER 13

The Woman and Her Voice

"A little bitty soft weensy voice makes you feel little bitty soft and weensy."[1]

The modern woman receives much conflicting advice about her voice. She also has conflicting voice models. While she may admire the low-pitched, seductive voice of Lauren Bacall, her voice in professional situations may require the persistent, inquiring sound of someone like Barbara Walters. A woman may find that her voice varies according to how much she has spoken and the situation in which she finds herself, and that it is heavily influenced by her physical health. As the quotation above suggests, the voice a woman uses often contributes to the way she feels about herself. The modern woman, like her male counterpart, is best off when she finds her natural voice and uses it in most situations.

In this chapter, we will take a look at the female voice from before puberty through old age. We will consider the physical factors, primarily hormonal, that heavily influence the sound of the female voice. We will then look at some of the social factors in modern society that shape the way women sound. And, finally, we will offer specific suggestions that can help most women find and maintain their natural voices in the various situations in which they find themselves: at work, home, and play.

The Female Voice

We all know that an adult female voice is higher in pitch than an adult male voice of the same age. What we often do not appreciate, how-

[1] Stone, J., and Bachman, J. (1977). *Speaking up.* New York: McGraw-Hill, p. 23.

ever, is that the female voice pitch also drops markedly as girls go through puberty. At age 9, boys and girls have the same voice pitch (around 265 Hz or slightly above middle C on the musical scale). During puberty the female speaking voice drops three or four musical notes. By age 20, a common pitch level for young adult women is an A below middle C (near 220 Hz). As we seen in Figure 13-1, the female voice pitch generally lowers slightly over the life span. (For further details about pitch changes, you might wish to review the early sections of Chapter 7, The Well-Aimed Pitch.)

As women grow older, their pitch level gets lower. Their voices can also get rougher at times, as you can see by the crosshatches on the pitch line in Figure 13-1. This vocal roughness, we generally call hoarseness.

FIGURE 13-1. Female voice changes over time.

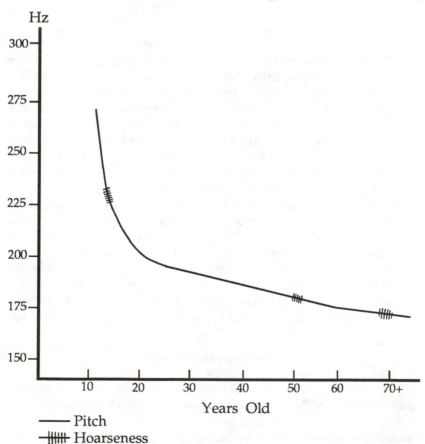

Some girls experience mild hoarseness during their early teenage years. If they are also high school cheerleaders, they may experience more hoarseness caused by their forced yelling. This vocal roughness will usually disappear during their 20s, 30s, and 40s, giving the typical woman a clear, normal voice during the majority of her working years.

After the menopause, women typically experience some lowering of pitch, sometimes accompanied by a small amount of hoarseness, with each new decade of life. Fortunately, research studies in recent years suggest that older women who are physically fit seem to display the same clarity of voice as younger women.

Another prominent voice characteristic of the American woman is that her voice has a tendency to inflect upward toward the end of a sentence. This is in contrast to the typical male voice pattern, which characteristically drops downward at the end of a sentence. This upward inflectional shift appears to be culturally learned and projects an image of a more passive person. It also conveys an impression of unsureness. The more aggressive, classic male voice inflects down, conveying an image of confidence.

Unlike pitch and hoarseness characteristics that are physically caused, inflectional behaviors appear to be learned, and they generally follow the stereotypic model that one perceives as fitting for one's age, sex, and role. As we will see later in this chapter, voice inflection patterns can be changed to meet the self-image requirements of any particular situation.

Physical Causes of Voice Change in the Female

In this section we will look at physical changes that influence the voice of the normal woman. We will not consider vocal abnormalities and their causes, which have been mentioned in other chapters.

The human larynx is heavily influenced by hormonal changes. The female in particular seems to experience hormone-induced voice changes during particular times in her life, such as during puberty, menstruation, pregnancy, and the menopause.

The pubescent changes in the female larynx are well documented. With the increase of estrogen (female hormone), the cartilages and muscles of the larynx enlarge greatly in size. The vocal cords of a 10-year-old girl are about 10 mm long; at age 15, they have increased to the adult length of 14 to 17 mm. These changes in size contribute to the lowering of the girl's natural speaking voice. As you may remember from earlier chapters, voice pitch is directly related to the tension and size of the vocal cords. A young woman may also experience a small amount of hoarseness during her menstrual cycle.

While much has been written about the irritability, depression, fatigue, bloating, weight gain, and possible breast pain that can be part of the premenstrual syndrome, only in recent years have changes of voice been documented. Dr. Jean Abitbol and other physicians in Paris studied 38 female professional voice users between the ages of 21 and 40.[1] He found that 22 of them experienced premenstrual symptoms of hoarseness and vocal fatigue. Most of them experienced no voice difficulties later in the ovulation stage of their menstrual cycle.

Many investigators have found that the female vocal cords at the premenstrual time are often swollen with some water retention and vascular enlargement. Dr. Peifang Chen at the Shanghai Conservatory in China studied 69 female opera singers and found that 86 percent of them experienced premenstrual vocal symptoms related to vocal cord swelling.[2] She reported that this enlargement resulted in a slight lowering of voice pitch that was often accompanied by slight hoarseness.

These voice complaints are not anxiety-induced or psychogenic; they are caused by the physical changes of the vocal cords. For example, the loss of a note or two at the top of the singing range is well documented for female opera singers at premenstrual times. Consequently, most major opera companies today now have "grace days" built into their singers' contracts. A few days before their periods, female vocalists do not sing.

During the premenstrual period, women who use their voices a lot in their work should make a special effort to cut down vocal effort and try to use voice in as easy a manner as possible. Many of the suggestions in Chapter 15, Ten Easy Ways for Keeping a Natural Voice, will be helpful.

From age 20 through the late 40s, the voice of the normal woman holds up very well. There is a slight lowering of pitch over time, as we saw in Figure 13–1. Other than the mild vocal symptoms she may experience during the few premenstrual days, her voice is basically trouble free. Only if she is a heavy smoker or suffers from severe respiratory disease will she possibly experience voice problems that interfere with normal voice.

Despite the hormonal shifts experienced during most of pregnancy, effects on voice seem to be minor. From the seventh month on, however, the pregnant woman may find that the growing baby inside her interferes a bit with normal respiration. She might have to renew her breath more often, or say fewer words per breath.

Perhaps the biggest hormonal influence on the female voice comes during and after the menopause. Less estrogen is available, while at the same time there is some increase in the male hormone (testosterone), causing increased thickness of the membranes covering the vocal cords. There may also be some atrophy of the muscles of the larynx, and perhaps some calcification of the laryngeal cartilages. The post-menopausal woman also carries her larynx a bit lower in the neck. All of these physical changes seem to contribute to a continuing lowering of pitch level in advanced age.

The hoarseness that some older women also experience seems to occur only in women who undergo a general physical decline. Older women in good physical shape do not seem to show this hoarseness.

The typical older woman free of disease will probably have a normal, if lower, speaking voice. If she experiences a voice problem, some of the suggestions given later in this chapter for women of all ages may be of help.

Of some interest is the common finding that the speed of talking goes down with increasing age in both men and women. It takes older people longer to say the same passage than it does younger people. This slowing is perhaps directly caused by diminished breathing functions, such as lower lung volumes and reduced air pressures. This requires the older person to renew breath more often. Also, older people tend to prolong the vowels in the words they say (for reasons we do not know). This also contributes to fewer words said per minute.

The Social Aspects of Women's Voices

The American woman has made tremendous economic and social gains in the past 30 years. For the most part, her speaking voice has served her well as she has taken on professional and administrative responsibilities that previously belonged to males in such diverse fields as industry, banking, transportation, medicine, or law.

The majority of working women are married and have children. Unlike the husband, whose primary focus in life is more often his work, the typical female makes definitive role changes from her role in the workplace to her roles of wife and mother. These role shifts are accompanied by changes in voice, and here is where some vocal difficulties can occur.

In the voice clinic, we recently saw a 31-year-old sales executive, Lori, who was experiencing hoarseness and pain in her throat that appeared to be related to stress. Her day began early in the morning when she got breakfast for her lawyer husband and two children, ages 2 and 4. No one spoke much at that time, and when Lori spoke it was usually to hurry the children along so she could leave them at a day-care center and still make it to her office by eight o'clock.

As the chief executive of a 22-person office and sales staff, she used her voice all day long. She used what she considered "a voice of authority," which was lower in pitch and much louder than the voice she used at home. On the office telephone, she used a gentler voice, only to return to the authoritarian voice with the next office appointment. By the nature of her work, her days were filled with tension, and this tension caused her to clear her throat a lot.

In the evening her husband picked up the children and they were usually home before Lori got there. Lori and her husband prepared dinner together while the children played in the playroom next to the kitchen. During dinner, and until the children went to bed, Lori spent much time disciplining the children, often with a high-pitched censuring voice. Finally, after the children were asleep, Lori and her husband had some time together, during which she spoke in an easy, natural voice.

The story of Lori could be replicated by many young working mothers. She was caught in three distinct roles: executive, mother, and wife. Unfortunately, she had learned to use a different voice in each role. The best thing we were able to do for Lori's voice problem was to show her ways to use her natural voice in all situations. This helped her greatly.

Because of the constantly changing vocal demands that women face, some women like Lori, who change vocal roles often during a day, can develop hoarseness, pain in the throat, loss of voice volume, vocal fatigue, and sometimes complete loss of voice.

A good speaker, male or female, makes it look easy. Normal voice takes a minimum of effort. We have all heard women's voices that seemed to be produced with little or no effort. They are pleasant voices and are easy to listen to, perhaps similar to these four famous voices:

Margaret Thatcher. Regardless of what we might think about her politics, her voice is attractive.

Joan Lunden. A television personality who keeps a feminine grace with a strong, easy to listen to voice.

Barbara Bush. The clear voice and lower pitch of an older woman. Her voice always sounds friendly and produced without effort.

Betty White. This veteran television actress keeps a clear, youthful sounding voice. Also, she has a friendly voice to hear.

Some women's voices are less pleasant than those mentioned above. Usually they are produced with too much effort. Once again if we look at the voices of some well known people we can find some examples. They usually sound as if they are working extra hard to get their voices out:

Bette Davis. This wonderful actress always had an interesting voice. Her hoarseness, her abrupt way of speaking became her trademark.

Ann Landers. This talented columnist has a harsh and nasal voice. People who know her column well are always surprised when they first hear her on television.

Debra Norville. Within the same two-hour Today program, this interviewer uses several voice styles: a soft, easy voice contrasted with an abrasive, rising pitch and a hard, crisp speaking style.

Bea Arthur. This television actress with her great flair for comedy often seems to have a hoarse voice. At times, she appears to speak at the very bottom of her pitch range, which makes her voice sound strained.

There are good and bad voices all around us. If we develop an awareness of them, we can set better goals for our own voices.

Common Problems of the Female Voice

As we will see in the last section of this chapter, searching for and maintaining one's natural voice is the key to avoiding voice problems. The voice of a woman (like the voice of anyone) should mirror how she really feels inside. Since our inner feelings are always changing, the normal voice is always changing. Some voice change for different situations is to be expected.

The voice becomes a problem when the sound of the voice and the way it is produced interfere with communication. The way you sound may be telling your listeners something different than the words you are saying. You may sound angry when inside you do not feel that way. Or your voice may sound as if you are unsure of yourself while inside you are fully confident of what you are doing. And sometimes using a certain voice style can mask some of the emotions you may be experiencing. Let us look at some voice styles that carry particular images to our listeners.

Excessive Use of Low Pitch

Many women think it is attractive to use the lowest speaking pitch they can produce. Some feel this carries an authoritative sound that helps them sound as if they are in control of a situation. Some women think there are advantages to sounding like men, much to the irritation of many of their male listeners, often not realizing that their natural voices may give them better control. Some women think the low-pitched voices of Lauren Bacall and Bea Arthur are sexy and seductive. Interestingly, however, such low-pitched voices are not heard often in younger women under the age of 30.

There is probably no voice behavior harder on the larnyx than speaking too low. Speaking at the bottom of one's pitch range seems to cause the voice to lose its natural resonance. It sounds strained. It is difficult to hear. And what is worse, over time, the excessively low-pitched voice can lead to vocal cord pathology.

Using Hard Glottal Attack

As described in earlier chapters, hard glottal attack is speaking with exact precision, with each word sounding separated from other words. Such a voice replaces the normal speaking legato with a crisp staccato. Each word seems to require separate voicing. Bette Davis' voice was a classic example of abrupt glottal attack. Some female administrators use hard glottal attack to control the people around them.

Such a voice is hard to listen to over time. The woman who uses such a crisp attack is signaling her listeners: "I know what I'm talking about — don't you dare challenge me!" Obviously, such a speaking style is viewed as aggressive by many listeners. Such precise speech also makes listening difficult. Over time this crisp speaking style can lead to tissue changes (contact ulcers) on the back part of the vocal cords.

Using Heavy Word Stress

Far more female than male radio-television newscasters use exaggerated word stress. By word stress we mean saying a syllable or a word in a higher pitch, a bit louder, and often stretching out the word (prolonging the vowels). In listening to a tape of a female newscaster commenting on the abortion ruling by the Supreme Court, I heard these words stressed (in caps):

It is TIME for the women of AMERica, the PRIMary conSUMers in this NATion, to STAND UP for what IS their BAsic right.

Such continuous word stress defeats the purpose of stress, which is to highlight an occasional word within the sentence. It is hard on one's listeners, yet it is commonly used by broadcasters on local and national television. In everyday life, we do not hear too many women speak this way. When we do, they are usually in some kind of leadership role where the use of word stress is equated in their minds with aggressiveness and authority.

Speaking Too Softly

Many women complain that they are often not heard, particularly by their male co-workers. This is particularly common among women whose voices are low-pitched with an obvious focus in their throats. Other women continue to use the same voice loudness, whether they are speaking to one person or to a group of people.

The person who speaks too softly is often viewed by listeners as shy, timid, and perhaps feeling inferior. Just by speaking louder, these perceptions can change quite favorably for the speaker.

Voice Tips for the Female Adult

There is a diversity of roles for women today, and each perhaps requires some individualization of voice style. Some women love the role of being single, with all of the opportunities and restrictions that such a life brings. Others prefer the traditional role of homemaker and mother. Many women combine the roles of worker, mother, and wife. Others, as single parents, work to support their children. Some women prefer the challenge of executive and professional work situations, making their careers the primary focus of their lives. Obviously, for the female adult, there is no one voice for everyone and for every situation. Certainly there will be situations where some special use of voice is needed. For example, there may be times when you are unsure of a solution to a problem but it is important that you mask this unsureness from the people around you.

It does appear, however, that over the long haul most women will experience the best voice by trying to keep their natural voices, regardless of the situation in which they find themselves. The earlier chapters in this book that talked about respiration, loudness, pitch, focus, and nasality have relevance for every woman seeking to find and improve her natural voice. The tips below will help you develop voice control in particular situations.

Keep Your Pitch Where It Ought to Be

Throughout this book, we have talked about using a speaking pitch that is a few notes above your lowest pitch. Avoid speaking too low or too high. A 38-year-old female surgeon, Dr. B, began using the lowest pitched voice she could produce during her afternoon office hours. Apparently during her morning surgery schedule, she used a natural voice and experienced no problems. But by using her low-pitched voice all afternoon, by five o'clock, Dr. B's voice was reduced to a whisper. Speaking very long at the bottom of your pitch range can play havoc with the voice.

Don't be afraid to use a lower voice now and then to fit a particular situation, but don't make the mistake of using this low pitch all the time. Authority can be added to your voice just by dropping your voice pitch toward the end of a phrase or sentence. Most of the time, keep your pitch up where it ought to be. And remember, avoid speaking in a monotone by developing good pitch variability.

Keep a Good Oral Focus to Your Voice

Maintain the imagery of placing your voice right off the surface of your tongue in the center of your mouth. This will avoid the "eensy weensy" baby voice that comes from having the tongue too far forward. It will also avoid the country bumpkin voice caused from back tongue carriage. Most importantly, it will keep the focus of your voice out of your throat.

A voice with good oral focus is a healthy voice. There are very few hoarse voices with good oral focus. A focused voice will last all day, despite various vocal demands placed on it. It will produce a voice that people around you find easy to hear.

Change Your Loudness to Fit the Situation

There is no voice more boring than one that always uses the same pitch and loudness. At home with a child or a husband is an excellent place to play with the loudness of your voice. Like the whisper, save the moderately loud voice for certain situations. Whenever possible, avoid shouting (substitute a whistle or a bell for yelling at the kids).

In the work setting, it is important to vary the loudness of your voice for certain situations. Bonnie, who was a telephone receptionist, sounded fine on the phone but used the same loudness level with people who stopped at her desk. No one could hear her. Noisy occupations, such as working as an airline cabin attendant or on an assembly line, require one to speak in a louder voice to overcome the constant background noise.

Use More Downward Pitch Inflections

The upward pitch inflection at the end of a sentence denotes a question or unsureness. The voice of authority is usually characterized by a dropping inflection at the end of the sentence. As mentioned earlier in this chapter, women in most cultures tend to use more rising inflections than men do. This may be why, according to recent communication research, men "one-up" what women say, and often interrupt them. The rising inflection may be a signal for the man (or the other person) to begin speaking.

In any case, become aware of the power of inflections at the end of sentences. For the woman who wants more command in her voice, dropping her voice a note or two towards the end of the sentence will usually give her voice more authority.

Change Your Glottal Attack to Fit the Situation

Like pitch and loudness changes, occasional use of hard glottal attack can give more emphasis to what you are saying. But hard glottal attack should be reserved for those few situations where you need to make a point. Avoid sounding like some television newscasters who use hard glottal attack for almost every word they say. Continuous use of hard glottal attack gives unneeded emphasis and can be very irritating to listeners.

Use a soft-voice attack now and then. The soft glottal attack in Southern speech sounds as if it takes very little effort. It's easy to listen to. Use soft attack during easy, relaxed moments and feel how relaxing it can be to speak this way. The actress Joanne Woodward, whose early years were spent in Mississippi, still shows traces of easy glottal attack and is a good model for such an easy voice.

Use Word Stress for Occasional Emphasis

Word stress is giving particular words or syllables more voicing emphasis. Stressed words and syllables can be higher in pitch, louder, and/or more prolonged than normal.

For women who are in a position of authority, occasional use of word stress can be very useful. But save word stress for the few words that are truly important. Excessive use of word stress can work against you, often making you sound too aggressive and too self-important. Avoid sounding like the woman we mentioned earlier who stressed every third word or syllable. Such speech can become meaningless, as well as irritating.

Find a Few Voice Role Models
to Emulate (and Stay Away from)

Most of us have people whom we admire — athletes, actresses, politicians, your sister, or the woman next door. Make a list of people whose voices you like to hear and of those whose voices you do not like to hear. I made up lists of good and poor voices in the last section. Picking a voice model is a highly individualized task. What I like, or dislike, in a voice might be quite different from what you like or dislike. Neither of us is right or wrong. We each have our own internal models.

Take some time to listen to voices in your home and office, on television, in church, or in the store. Select four or five of the best voices. What is it that you like about them? Easy to listen to? Pitch? Quality? Sincerity? Now select four or five of the poorest voices you have heard. What is it about these voices that turns you off? Are they too loud, brash, grating, nasal, or any of the other negative voice descriptors from Chapter 1?

Now go back and listen to your own voice on a tape. See if you can find the qualities in your own voice that you like in other voices. You can build upon these by following some of the suggestions in this book. If you hear qualities in your voice that you don't like, see if you can eliminate them. Sometimes your ability to compare a good voice model to your own voice is the most important step in helping you improve your voice.

Finding one's natural voice and using it in most talking situations will give most women the voice they want — and deserve.

References

1. Abitbol, J., and others. (1989). Does a hormonal vocal cord cycle exist in women? *Journal of Voice, 3,* 157-162
2. Chen, Peifang. Personal correspondance.

CHAPTER 14

The Man and His Voice

*"It's not enough to sound masculine.
You want to sound like the kind of man
people listen and respond to."*

Like his female counterpart, the modern American man has learned that his voice conveys a large part of his image to others. Often it is not what he says but how he says it that matters to his listeners. If his voice sends false and negative messages about him, sometimes a book like this is all he needs to help him. A man's natural voice generally sounds best in all circumstances, and is made with the least amount of effort. On those occasions when he needs a different voice, his natural voice is still the foundation voice, the "home base" for his speaking.

In this chapter we will look at the male voice from childhood through old age. We will consider the physical factors that distinguish men's voices from women's. We will examine the voice problems common to men. And, finally, we will offer suggestions to help men use their voices to their best advantage.

The Male Voice

As we all know, males speak in a lower pitch than females, except in early childhood (up to age 11) when there is little difference. In fact, 11-year-old girls generally will have slightly lower pitched voices than boys do because the female generally begins puberty several years earlier.

Puberty begins in most boys around the age of 10 with an increase of the male hormone testosterone and seems to last about four years. Voice change, however, usually does not begin until after the second year of puberty. By age 14 the male voice pitch has dropped nearly an octave, close to D below middle C (147 Hz).

During the last six months of puberty, about one-third of all boys experience temporary pitch breaks, caused by rapid laryngeal growth. These are normal and disappear entirely as the larynx completes its growth.

By age 18, the typical young man has the speaking voice of an adult male, near C below middle C (131 Hz). His voice pitch will gradually lower over the succeeding years (see Figure 14-1) until he is in his 70s. In his early 70s, pitch levels begin to rise slightly.

During the rapid adolescent voice changes, some boys may exhibit a slight hoarseness, although many do not. For most of their adult years the majority of men have clear voices, except when the voice is affected by things such as allergies, infections, or heavy smoking. However, a rougher voice may again appear after age 70, as shown in Figure 14-1. But recent studies have shown that older men who are physically fit seem free of the hoarseness that less physically fit men experience around that age.

As we noted in the last chapter, the normal male voice tends to inflect downward at the end of sentences and phrases whereas the female voice tends to inflect upward. The dropping inflection is associated with sureness, the rising inflection with uncertainty. Panels of listeners asked to evaluate tape recordings of voices generally rate speakers whose inflections fall at the end of sentences as "knowing what they are talking about."

These subjective responses seem to be the result of cultural conditioning, as are the inflection habits themselves. Pitch and voice quality are primarily determined by physical causes. But voice inflections and word stresses seem to be culturally determined, shaped by perceived social pressures.

Obviously it makes a great deal of difference to your efforts to control how you speak whether a particular voice characteristic is physically or culturally conditioned. Let us first look at the physical factors that affect the male voice.

Physical Causes of Voice Changes in the Male

Around age 10 boys and girls have similar sized vocal cords, about 10 mm long, and about the same thickness. Boy and girl singers at this age are usually both sopranos. With the coming of puberty, the male larynx doubles in size. The typical adult male develops vocal cords around 20 mm long.

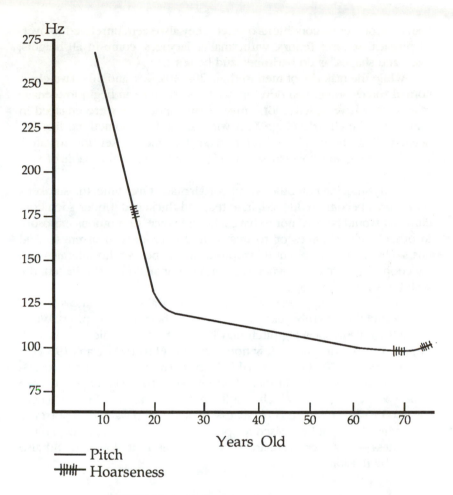

FIGURE 14-1. Male voice changes over time.

It is the influence of the male hormone testosterone that makes laryngeal growth so dramatic in men. The adult male larynx is also markedly different in composition than the adult female larynx, with more and larger striated muscle fiber, less tissue fat, and larger cartilages. It also becomes visually prominent, producing the bulge in the front of the neck that we call the Adams' apple. These longer, thicker vocal cords produce a voice that has dropped an octave from prepubertal levels, and generally is half an octave lower than a woman's voice.

Male larynges vary greatly in size from person to person, however. The differences appear to be related primarily to genetic factors, rather than environmental conditions or diet. They also seem unrelated to over-all physical stature. Tenors, with smaller larynges, come in all heights, sizes, and shapes, as do baritones and basses.

While the majority of men in their 20s, 30s, 40s, and 50s have clear, normal voices, some men develop hoarseness. This can begin in teenage years if they have yelled a lot while playing sports, or were engaged in something like cheerleading. With vocal abuse from something like frequent yelling, the vocal cord membranes become thicker and irritated. The thickening and hoarseness often goes away when the habit of yelling stops.

Heavy smoking is another vocal cord irritant. Over time, the smoker's vocal cords become reddened, irritated, and thickened. Under such conditions it would be hard not to have a hoarse voice. Continuous exposure to other kinds of fumes or to dust can also produce hoarseness. And hoarseness is also a common symptom of our bouts with allergies and infections. In these cases, when the source of irritation is eliminated, the symptoms usually disappear.

There is a slight, progressive increase in vocal cord thickness among men during their mature years, which lowers their speaking pitch. While at age 20 a man's speaking pitch may be at C below middle C (131 Hz), by age 50 it has dropped a few notes to an A (110 Hz) or a G (98 Hz).

Around age 70, the hormonal balance between estrogen and testosterone begins to change in men. Consequently, the male begins to lose some vocal cord tissue, which results in a slight raising of pitch. There can also be some increased hoarseness. An actor who wanted to portray a man in his 90s might be advised to speak in a higher voice and add a bit of hoarseness — a Walter Brennan voice. Speaking a bit slower could also add to the illusion.

The Social Aspects of Men's Voices

Men's and women's voices remain distinct in contemporary society, despite the occasional androgynous rock star and unisex fashions. Nor have changes in the relations between the sexes in the workplace, socially, and in the home produced a tendency for men and women to speak like one another. Indeed, as we saw in the previous section, physical factors would make this impossible, even if men or women found it desirable.

Women who have moved into positions that were traditionally held exclusively by men sometimes try to alter the way they speak in certain situations, perhaps to sound more authoritative. But this is a matter of changing patterns of stress and inflection, not the basic feminine characteristics of their voices.

Although men have not noticeably tried to feminize their voices, even when they work largely with or for women, some men may try to sound even more masculine in such situations. Others make some effort to soften the way they speak around women (many men have long done this socially) from the more aggressive speaking manner they normally use in strictly male company.

What men have in common with women in an era of changing sex roles is voice problems related to having to use many different voices during the day. Jerry, the owner of a busy restaurant in a California resort city, is a good example. At home in the morning he liked to wrestle and romp with his two children, and make lots of funny noises to amuse them. With the children off to school, he changed to a softer, caring voice with his wife before he went to work. When he reached the restaurant, at the beginning of a hectic lunch hour, he was instantly in high gear, using a louder, higher pitched voice to be heard over the clatter of glasses and dishes, the buzz of conversation, and the restaurant's background music. He also altered his voice depending on whom he was talking to. He had a tough voice when he talked to the kitchen help and his busboys, a coaxing voice when he talked to some of his attractive waitresses, and a smooth, accommodating voice when he spoke to some of his steady customers. After the lunch hour rush, Jerry might have some minutes of quiet conversation with those customers, or he could be yelling, on the telephone or in person, at some supplier who had failed to deliver what the restaurant needed for that night or the next day.

His afternoon was slow. At home, or on his sailboat in fine weather, Jerry and his wife talked quietly of their plans for the future, or sometimes more earnestly of business problems. In the evening the restaurant was even more of a madhouse than at lunch time. By the time Jerry said goodnight to his wife in the small hours of the morning, often the only voice he had left was a tiny croak.

It was his wife who suggested Jerry come to us, when the good night croak began to show up in the daytime too. "He used to have such a pleasant voice," she said, "almost like a television announcer's. Now he sounds as if he's swallowed a rasp and is mad at me and everyone else."

We were able to help Jerry by first helping him to find his natural voice, and then teaching him how to use it as the foundation for the voices he needed to cope with the wide variety of speaking circumstances he faced every day. Jerry found that his natural voice came out easily, with little effort, and still accomplished what he needed to accomplish in his work.

We hear good and bad voices around us every day. A good voice is usually one that seems appropriate to the speaker's age and sex, and to the circumstances he or she has to deal with. At the same time it is distinctively the speaker's own. It is always easy to produce and does not over-tax the vocal equipment.

Public figures often have developed such voices. Consider a few.

Gregory Peck. Over the years most of us have been impressed with his deep resonant voice. It projects an image of sureness.

Johnny Carson. You never think about Johnny's voice. It is just there, pleasant, but attention-getting. He always keeps an excellent voice focus.

Tom Cruise. His is a youthful voice, natural, clear, and always at the right pitch level for a person in his late-twenties.

James Earl Jones. This fine actor has a beautifully resonant voice. Although he has a deep pitch, he keeps absolute oral focus. His is probably one of the most outstanding voices in this country.

Many men's voices are distinctively different from the way most men talk. In some cases, what is bad about such voices may be responsible for a good deal of the person's public image and success. Because of that we tend to think of their voices as different rather than bad. The four men listed below have different voices with qualities that could be considered bad.

Harry Belafonte. While his singing voice is hauntingly beautiful, it is difficult to listen to his persistently hoarse speaking voice.

George Bush. The President's distinctive voice has a high pitch and a little too much front focus. He prolongs his vowels for emphasis on certain words.

Michael Jackson. This very popular singer has quite a high speaking pitch, low volume, and is often hoarse.

George Burns. His hoarse voice has been part of his radio and television image for the past 50 years. Because of his hoarseness, he cannot speak loudly enough for some people to hear him comfortably.

You can probably add some good and bad male speaking voices to these lists. If you develop an awareness of the qualities that make them good or bad you can set better goals for your own voice. Keep in mind that it is your *natural* voice that you are looking for, not a celebrity voice, or a voice that is different just for the sake of sounding different.

Common Problems of the Male Voice

A natural voice is one produced in a way that will not cause voice problems to develop. Unfortunately, men tend to abuse their vocal mechanisms more than women do, and so problems appear frequently. Let us look at some of the problems common to the adult male.

Inappropriate Use of Pitch

Some men, and some women, believe that the male image is enhanced by speaking in as low a pitch as possible. But speaking at the bottom of one's pitch range requires a lot of muscle tension. As a result the voice can sound strained and lack resonance. Moreover, the low-pitched voice often has a low sounding focus, coming from deep down in the throat, which makes it difficult to hear in noisy situations.

Perhaps because the social penalties are too great, relatively few men speak in a high pitch. But some do, and this can strain the vocal equipment too. Finding and using your natural pitch, as shown in Chapter 7, is a good way to overcome problems of too-low or too-high pitch.

Inappropriate Loudness Levels

Men frequently work in noisier environments than women do. Not only can this create voice strain from trying to speak over the noise all day, but many men also use the same loud voice when they leave the job.

Men are usually noisier in their play than women, in their sports and on social occasions. One of the ways men seem to assert their masculinity is by talking louder. Listen to a group of teenagers practicing being macho by raising their voices or to a group of men watching a ball game at a stadium or a bar.

Men also use a louder voice as a way of controlling people around them, whether at work, play, or in the home. The man who does this frequently is the man who does not adjust his loudness for different situations — loudness is a hard thing for him to relinquish.

Other men talk too softly, so softly they are hard to understand, and they can project an image of timidity, particularly in all-male surroundings. Soft talkers can have a physical problem, perhaps respiratory or neurological, that makes it impossible for them to speak any louder. But usually they talk softly out of long habit, for reasons that have to do with their overall personality. The habitual soft-talker, like the habitual loud-talker, does not adjust his voice volume for the circumstances he is in.

Loudness adjustment, however, is a key to being heard and understood. The soft talker might not be heard. The loud-talker might not be understood, or might be resented, and so his message is ignored. Chapter 6 showed you how to adjust the loudness of your voice so that it is appropriate to the circumstances you are in.

Yelling

Some men love to yell. Yelling should be avoided because it is so hard on the voice, but that is not always possible. In certain types of industrial plants and on construction sites, men often have to communicate by yelling, and that is certainly true in many competitive sports. In all of these situations communication is important, but when they have to yell many men do so in a low-pitched voice. This is hard to hear in noisy situations, and it is hard on the voice.

A star NFL quarterback had that problem at the beginning of his professional career. He had difficulty making his signals heard. Particularly when his team was on the road, at enclosed arenas such as Seattle's Kingdome, his team couldn't hear the plays he called over the crowd noise. The quarterback felt that several games had been lost because of this. We found that when he tried to bark out his signals it was in the gruffest, loudest voice he could produce. Once he was taught to yell in a higher pitched voice with good mouth focus, his play-calling could be heard in any but the most raucous crowd noise — and his voice lasted for all four quarters too.

To protect the voice, as well as keep it understandable, men who must yell should take in bigger breaths, say fewer words, and use a higher pitch with good oral focus.

Throat Focus

Men are more apt than women to speak with low throat focus, from deep back in their throats. This can produce a voice that is hoarse and hard to hear. Throughout this book we have pointed out that the best sounding voice sounds as if it comes right off the surface of your tongue and in the middle of your mouth.

We have also found that good focus is somewhat independent of pitch. That is, you can have a low-pitched voice and still have high mouth focus. In Chapter 8, and later in this chapter, we will tell you some easy ways to develop better oral focus.

Pitch Breaks

Upward pitch breaks are embarrassing to men who have them. We are not talking about the pitch breaks experienced by some adolescent boys, which disappear with maturity. We speak of adult men whose voices occasionally break upward. If they gave an order, it might sound like

I told you to get off the fence

with the two marked words breaking up an octave from the regular pitch.

Fortunately, such a problem is easy to correct. All the man has to do is raise his regular speaking voice one or two notes and the pitch breaks usually disappear. Upward pitch breaks in men are usually caused by habitually speaking at a pitch level that is too low and is produced with some strain. The voice escapes this uncomfortable range from time to time by breaking upward. A slight raising of your customary pitch gets rid of the problem.

Singing the Wrong Part

Many of us sing from time to time, in a church choir, glee club, or community theater musical, as well as in informal gatherings of friends. Singing can be harmful to a man's voice if he sings the wrong part — and this can happen even in more formally organized groups. Choral music frequently is divided into four parts: soprano and alto for women, tenor and bass for men. Often it does not include a part for baritones, even though that is the normal singing range for most men. The result is that men are often forced to sing higher as tenors or lower as basses.

After an extended stretch of this, the tenor or bass who is really a baritone may have throat dryness and pain. He may even find that he has difficulty speaking in his regular voice range and is hoarse. These symptoms disappear as if by magic by not singing the *extremes* of the singing part, avoiding the highest notes of the tenor range or the lowest notes of the bass range. If you are singing with an organized group, consultation with the singing director, or with a singing teacher, can be helpful. If you are singing more informally, be alert to the symptoms we noted above, and take the necessary steps to ease the problem.

Voice Tips for the Adult Male

As is true for women, men's voices are called on for a variety of roles in work, social, and family life. For men who are salesmen, lawyers, and teachers, voice is vital to their livelihood. In occupations like farming and research the voice is used far less. But all of us need our voices to represent us well some of the time at work, and it is always important socially or at home.

While most men would profit from using their natural voice in most situations, there are times when, temporarily, they need to sound a little different. For example, a judge annoyed by the performance of a lawyer in court cannot always afford the luxury of letting that annoyance show in his voice. (Even less can a lawyer let his voice show that he is annoyed with a judge!) But all men face circumstances when they do not want their voices to betray their feelings, or when they need their voices to convey a little more conviction or authority.

Let us look at some things that men can do to better control the way they sound.

Use Pitch and Pitch Changes to Get Your Message Across

You can add authority to your voice by lowering your pitch level. This should be done sparingly. If you always speak at the bottom of your pitch range, it is impossible to inflect your voice any lower when you want to add some authority. If you keep it too low you also run the risk of pitch breaks.

A man comfortable with himself will use rising inflections now and then. Pitch elevation at the end of occasional sentences will encourage your listeners to speak up, ask questions, and so you develop a better rapport with them.

Use Loudness and Loudness Changes for Emphasis

There is nothing more boring than listening to someone give (or read!) a speech in the same monotonous voice, never varying his loudness. Or the man who always talks in a loud voice who sounds boorish and intimidating. His voice is saying, "I'm talking! Don't interrupt!" or "I'm the only one with all the answers."

On the other hand, a man who always speaks softly is often viewed as timid and unsure of himself. Although he may have a lot to say, what he says may not always be heard. A good guideline is to speak as loudly as the people around you. A soft-spoken person needs to take in slightly larger breaths and say fewer words per breath. Like the habitual loud-talker, he needs to be careful not to sound monotonous and he needs to vary his loudness. Chapter 6 can help men who need better control over the loudness of their voices.

Keep the Right Focus to Your Voice

Pay close attention to well-focused voices like those of Paul Newman, Harrison Ford, Ed McMahan, Walter Cronkite, and Peter Jennings.

Regardless of what pitch they use, their voices always sound as if focus is in their mouths. They are easy to hear and easy to understand.

Although the most common voice focus problem of men is a voice that sounds as if it comes from way back in the throat, a few men have voices too far forward in focus. They sound the way Truman Capote did, with thin, effeminate speech. The problem can be corrected just by bringing the tongue a bit farther back. Men who have the problem of focus too far back in the throat can correct it by bringing the tongue a little forward when they speak. A little practice with tongue positions, using your tape recorder, will make these differences clear to you.

Further suggestions for developing good voice focus can be found in Chapter 8. The benefits of a well-focused voice are that it can always be heard, sounds better, and does not tire easily.

Change the Friendliness of Your Voice

There are times when we don't want to sound friendly, when an unfriendly voice may be necessary or useful — at least times when a friendly voice is simply inappropriate. A frown and a downturned mouth, the opposite of a smile, will color the sound of your voice. You can also show displeasure by lowering your pitch level and dropping your word inflections at the end of phrases and sentences with some finality.

But most of the time most of us want to sound friendly. Both at work and in our social lives we get more positive results when we do. The problem is that some men normally have unfriendly voices, particularly on the telephone. Without wanting to, or even being aware of it, they sound angry or irritated most of the time.

This can be helped in several ways. For one thing, smile more as you talk. Research studies show that people listening to taped voices can tell whether or not the speaker was smiling. The act of smiling influences the sound of the voice — try it with your tape recorder and you will hear the difference. Laughter does the same thing. It seems to open up the throat and relax the voice, making the speaker sound more friendly and less fearful. We often encourage laughter for our patients who have severe tight voices.

You will also sound friendlier when you feel happy inside. Take a moment before speaking to someone to reflect on your mood. Often we are basically happier than we allow ourselves to think we are (if we think of it at all). Let it show in your voice. You'll speak faster and often with some humor.

Listen to your regular voice on tape. Do you sound like a friendly person? If you do, fine — remember that sound. If you don't, but you want to, try some of the above suggestions.

Using Rising Voice Inflections to Include Others in Conversation

Many men talk too much. Competitive as we are, we try to dominate the conversation in groups and don't always take the time to let others talk, or to listen to them when they do.

Healthy, normal conversation is a two-way affair: we talk–we listen, we talk–we listen. By using low pitch, loudness, and falling inflections, many men control conversation instead. It may do something for their egos, or anxieties, but it is not true conversation, and it often stirs up resentment and resistance among listeners.

A lot of men control conversations this way just out of habit. They have become insensitive to the fact that each conversational situation requires a different approach. Or they simply don't know how to help create a conversation in which all parties participate.

An obvious way to get listener participation is by directly asking questions of others. Rising vocal inflections at the ends of phrases and sentences also invite listeners to respond with their ideas. If we couple this with a smiling face, the invitation is even clearer (and it is friendly).

You can experiment with the technique using your tape recorder. Try reading or improvising some sentences that you might normally use in your work, but give rising inflections to the ends of phrases or sentences where you want to encourage listener participation. Don't forget to pause a bit, so they have time to speak up. And don't overdo it, so you sound as if you're unsure of yourself. That is where a smile can really help. A slight rising inflection along with a smile clearly signals that you want to hear from your listeners. You'll be able to hear it on the tape.

Men, as well as women, will find that using their natural voices in the various roles they are called on to play will give them the best sounding voice, and the most effective one. In situations when circumstances require them to play a particular part, a different voice may be required temporarily. There are techniques for doing that, too, as we have shown.

By this point in the book you have found your natural voice, your natural breathing, loudness, pitch, and focus, and you have learned something about using it even in special or difficult circumstances. It is time now to give you the techniques to maintain your natural voice so that it is always there for you to use when you want it.

CHAPTER **15**

Ten Easy Steps for Keeping Your Natural Voice

"A good maintenance program for your natural voice is neither difficult nor time consuming."

Today most of us are aware that taking care of our health involves more than going to see a doctor when we don't feel well. Millions now follow some regular exercise program and are careful about how much and what foods they eat. We have learned that there is a great deal we can do ourselves to keep healthy.

A healthy, natural voice benefits from the same kind of awareness and attention. Now that you have corrected some of the problems you have had with your voice, and have learned to use your natural voice, you can easily keep it that way by following the maintenance program in this chapter. It is neither difficult nor time consuming. All you need to do is use this chapter from time to time as a reminder and review.

Use your tape recorder, which was so helpful in many of the previous tests and exercises, to record a few minutes of both conversation and reading. Then listen critically to the tape.

The Voice Checklist (see Table 15-1) can help you see whether each dimension of your voice is where you want it to be. Listen to your tape and rate yourself 1 through 7 on each dimension. A *normal* or natural rating on the Voice Checklist is a 4. *Extreme problems* of voice on the scale would be a 1 or 7. Most of the time, if we still find we have a problem with voice, the problem is *slight* (a 3 or 5 on the scale) or *moderate* (a 2 or 6 rating).

TABLE 15-1. The Voice Checklist

Voice Dimension	Ratings						
Breathing (words per breath)	1 Too Few	2	3	4 Normal	5	6	7 Too Many
Loudness	1 Soft	2	3	4 Natural	5	6	7 Too Loud
Pitch	1 Low	2	3	4 Natural	5	6	7 High
Pitch inflections	1 None	2	3	4 Normal	5	6	7 Excessive
Horizontal focus	1 Back	2	3	4 Normal	5	6	7 Front
Vertical focus	1 Throat	2	3	4 Normal	5	6	7 Nasal
Nasality	1 Denasal	2	3	4 Balanced	5	6	7 Hypernasal
Hoarseness	1 Breathy	2	3	4 Normal Quality	5	6	7 Harsh Tight

Any of the voice problems mentioned in this book can range from slight to severe. Throughout the book, for purposes of illustration, we have usually talked about severe cases. In reality, most of our voice problems are more likely to be slight or moderate problems with breathing, loudness, pitch, focus, or nasality. If you have rated yourself different than normal on any items of the Voice Checklist, you will probably want to go back and review the chapter dealing with that particular problem, and do the exercises suggested until the problem has been eliminated.

Whether your voice problem is only slight or occasional, however, it is still a problem that needs attention. First of all, you want to always sound your best. Second, some slight voice problems have a way of developing into severe ones, and some occasional problems into permanent ones. Third, even if that is not the case, a slight problem can draw a negative reaction from your listeners. Think of a voice with slight nasality or denasality, or a voice that is always slightly too loud or too soft, too high or low in pitch.

If you have given yourself 4s, or normal scores, on all of the items, good for you. That is what we designed this book to do, to enable you to find and use your natural voice consistently, to present yourself, through your voice, as the person you really are.

But even if you have no voice problem, you can greatly benefit from a regular program of natural voice maintenance, from staying aware of those things that are most helpful and most harmful to good voice.

Just as you may keep in your kitchen a list of healthy and unhealthy food ingredients, or a reminder on your closet door of exercises you want to perform each day, you many want to keep the list that follows, Ten
Easy Steps for Keeping Your Natural Voice, in some handy place.

The 10 steps have been presented many times before in this book. Here we group them all together for convenient review. They are hints that will enable you to keep your natural voice regardless of the situation in which you find yourself.

Ten Easy Steps for Keeping Your Natural Voice

1. Cut Down on Throat Clearing and Coughing. Don't Yell.

Many potentially good voices are destroyed by vocal abuse. Three of the most common abuses are throat clearing, coughing, and yelling.

Throat clearing is hard on the voice, and is often more a habit than a necessity. When you clear your throat, you may raise a small amount of mucous but the act bangs the vocal cords together unnecessarily and can cause some tissue irritation. The irritated mucosal tissue then exudes its own mucous. The process becomes self-generating: The more you clear your throat, the more you need to do so.

Habitual throat clearers need to make a conscious effort to curb the habit. One way to do it is to sniff with intensity as a substitute for clearing the throat. This quick sniff can rid the vocal cords of some mucous and we then swallow what we sniff.

Another way to clear your throat is to do it as silently as you can. Silent throat clearing is much less irritating to the vocal cords.

Continous heavy coughing is also hard on the vocal cords. High-speed photography of the larynx during a cough shows that the vocal cords slam together and are blown apart suddenly by the outgoing air. As a result of this trauma, continued heavy coughing can result in swollen, irritated vocal cords, which make normal voice almost impossible.

Often there is a physical cause for continuous coughing, such as a bad cold, an allergy, or smoke. Such conditions require medical treatment. Some coughing, however, becomes a habit, just as throat clearing does. For this kind of habit we need to practice the "silent cough," coughing as silently as we can. The silent cough is far easier on the vocal cords than the loud cough we usually make.

Yelling is another vocal practice that is very hard on the voice, and we need to avoid yelling whenever possible. Except in rare emergencies, most yelling is not necessary.

If you must yell on occasion, do it sensibly. Use a lot of breath behind your voice, a higher pitch, and good mouth focus. This will enable your voice to carry with better volume. Still, if you want to keep a better voice, the less you yell the better.

2. Develop an Easy Voice Attack (Use Southern Speech)

Voice attack is related to the degree of abruptness with which we say our words. In music, this easy attack is called *legato,* where there are no discernible breaks between notes. In voice, an easy attack blends words and sounds together gently, as in Southern speech. We hear that easy voicing in voices like Jimmy Carter's or Joanne Woodward's. A hard, abrupt attack can be heard in many Northeastern voices, such as those of Don Adams, Bette Davis, or Howard Cosell.

The soft, legato-like voice is a lot easier on the vocal cords — and on the ears of our listeners. Hard voice attack takes too much effort. The larynx tires easily and the vocal cords can become irritated from such continuous abrupt usage.

Between talking abruptly or with an easy voice attack, there is no contest. The easy voice sounds better and it doesn't strain or tire the larynx.

3. Use a Pitch Level That Is Natural for You.

Many men try to sound authoritative by speaking at the bottom of their pitch ranges. Some professional women attempt to sound more in command by speaking with too low a pitch. Other people use voices that are pitched too high. As we pointed out in Chapter 7, most of us will get better mileage out of our voices by using an average pitch level that is several notes above our lowest note.

When we talk about your best pitch level, we are speaking of the level that is easy and natural for you, the level you will probably use about 70 percent of the time when you speak. But none of us should have an absolute pitch level that we use all the time. Varying our pitch up and down as we stress particular words or syllables gives our voices inflections. It makes our speech livelier, more interesting, and avoids the dull monotone.

In Chapter 7 you found your natural pitch level. That is the baseline for your pitch, and it is the level at which you will usually sound your best.

4. Develop Good Vertical and Horizontal Focus for Your Voice.

Many people have voices that sound as if they come from deep in their throats. Other voices are focused too high in the nose and sound nasal. Still others are produced too far forward (the baby voice) or too far back (the Alf voice). A good, natural voice sounds as if it is focused right on the top of your tongue in the middle of your mouth. It is also an efficient voice and one that can stand up to a lot of use. A voice with good focus is durable and will always be there when you need it.

5. Renew Your Breath More Often By Pausing

Renewing your breath more often as you speak is important for keeping your natural voice and avoiding voice strain. Trying to speak without adequate air, by muscular exertion alone, is a real workout for the vocal tract.

There are two ways to develop good breathing habits while speaking. First, become aware of how many words you can easily say on one breath. If you frequently run out of air as you speak, try to use only a fraction (say one-half) of that number of words before you pause for breath.

Second, learn when to pause. There are natural breaks in what we say that easily permit a pause: before an important word (the pause preceding it gives it more emphasis), wherever there is a comma in a written text, and at the ends of phrases and sentences.

The pause provides you with an automatic renewal of breath. With a good breath supply behind your vibrating vocal cords, you should easily be able to maintain a good, natural voice.

6. Reduce Your Demands on Your Voice. Don't Do All the Talking.

Some voices are destroyed by overwork. To maintain a healthy, natural voice it is important to avoid excessive talking.

It has been my observation over the years that many of the people with voice problems have such gregarious personalities that they talk all the time. Friendly chattiness, and being the life of the party, is fine. But overdoing it can result in negative voice symptoms such as hoarseness or a voice that becomes weak or faint.

If those symptoms do appear, a conscious effort to cut down talking, or simply being quiet, will often help to renew a tired voice. Many people, however, have to use their voices a lot because of the kind of work they do. For them, the nine other vocal hygiene suggestions in this chapter can be of great help in maintaining the best possible voice under those conditions. A voice that is used a lot needs to be used properly.

7. Develop an Open Vocal Tract. Remember the Yawn-Sigh.

Many voices are destroyed by tightening of the vocal tract, by shutting down the larynx, the throat, and the mouth. A voice produced like that sounds tense and often lacks volume and normal resonance. There are several things that we can do to develop a more open, relaxed voice.

Keep your mouth open more. A slight opening of your lips, and a gentle opening (not much wider than the thickness of a pocket comb) between your upper and lower front teeth can contribute a great deal to developing an easy, relaxed voice.

An open vocal tract can be developed even when you are not talking. While you listen to someone else, or when you read or watch television, make a deliberate effort to keep your mouth slightly open.

Remember the yawn-sigh. No other vocal technique opens up a tight vocal tract as quickly as this one. The vocal tract opens maximally when we yawn. The yawn inhalation creates a wide open airway, and the exhaled sigh that follows produces a very relaxed voice, primarily because the vocal tract is still wide open. In any situation where your throat feels tense and your voice sounds tight, use the yawn-sigh.

8. Avoid Talking in Loud Settings. Watch the Noise Level.

Talking against a background of loud noise can strain anyone's voice. One of the noisiest backgrounds around is the modern disco. It can be so loud that people cannot monitor their own voices and end up shouting and adding to the general din. But nowadays even many bars and restaurants have not only a loud television set going but background music as well. After prolonged attempts to talk in such a setting, one often experiences symptoms of vocal fatigue, throat discomfort, and hoarseness.

Other settings where background noise can be a problem are less obvious. Conversing during a long car ride, on a commercial jet, or at a ball game can tax your voice. Talking above loud music at home, around power mowers or leaf blowers, or even when home or shop appliances are running can cause vocal fatigue.

If you must talk is such noisy places, your voice will last longer if you speak with a vertical focus and a slightly higher pitch level. And remember, the louder you speak the more air you need. At these louder levels, you should say fewer words between breaths.

9. Avoid Smoking and Excessive Use of Alcohol.

The person who needs to use his or her voice a lot, and wants to maintain a natural voice, should avoid smoking. The mucous membranes of the throat and vocal cords become inflamed and swollen from the dryness, heat, and tars from tobacco smoke. If you experience persistent hoarseness or other vocal problems as a result of smoking, a trial period of not smoking may be all that is needed to restore the voice to normal. Incidentally, marijuana smoke is a much hotter smoke than smoke from regular cigarettes and, therefore, a greater vocal cord irritant.

Mild (two drinks a day or less) or occasional use of alcohol seems to have no negative effects on the voice. Heavier daily use (three or more drinks), however, can have negative effects. Excessive alcohol dilates the tiny blood vessels on the vocal cords and can produce a lower pitch with some hoarseness — the voice of the well-known "whiskey tenor."

10. Watch Your Water Needs: Humidity and Liquids.

Excessive dryness is hard on the voice. I often tell my clients that "a healthy voice is a wet one." People who are concerned about their voices should pay attention to both the amount of liquid they drink and the dryness of the air they breathe. Excessive dryness can irritate the membranes covering the vocal cords and cause swelling. On examination of patients with excessively dry mouths, we also find some redness and red-streaking of the membranes of the back of the throat. Such irritation often is eliminated completely by drinking more fluids.

Certain medications can also have drying effects on the vocal tract. Antihistamines have an immediate drying effect. There are, however, antihistamines available that contain a moisturizer, an important help for those who must use their voice a lot but who have to take antihistamines. Drugs such as diuretics, often used for the treatment of high blood pressure, can also cause extensive dryness of the throat and larynx. People who take such medications should check with their doctors or pharmacists to see if the drug has a side effect of throat dryness. If dryness is a problem, sometimes another medication can be substituted.

The humidity of the air we breathe can affect how we sound. One reason that singers favor nose breathing is that air passing through the nose and throat becomes warmer and more moist. Some moisture in the air is essential for normal voice. Humidity under 20 percent, or over 50 percent, may require you to do something to change the moisture level in your environment.

Air conditioners and gas furnaces can remove much of the humidity from the air. Get a humidifier or vaporizer to replace it. In damp climates, air conditioners and dehumidifiers may be required to remove excess moisure in the air.

In follow-up studies of patients with voice problems, we have found that changing the humidity levels (higher or lower) in rooms where they live, sleep, or work can have positive effects in decreasing their negative voice symptoms.

This chapter is probably all that most of you will need in the future to maintain the good, natural voice that you have found with the help of this book. Rereading it from time to time will refresh your memory about the good voice habits you have learned, and about the bad habits you need to avoid.

The following chapter is intended primarily for those of you who have not been able to eliminate your voice problems. But it will also be of help for any user of voice who wants to know what professional help is available for particularly difficult or persistent voice problems.

CHAPTER **16**

Professional Help for Voice Problems

"My voice is still bad. What do I do now?"

After reading the previous chapters, you probably have developed a new awareness of your own voice and the voices around you. You have a more accurate idea of how you sound. You know what voice practices can give you a bad voice and what things you can do to develop a better, more natural voice. You probably also remember that a sudden change of voice, such as hoarseness that lasts for more than 10 days, despite what you do to improve it, should be investigated by a doctor.

This 10-day rule for sudden and continued hoarseness is a good one to remember. And although this book is about adult voice problems and voice improvement, the 10-day rule is particularly important to keep in mind for children, 16 years old and younger. Hoarseness in children can be a symptom of serious laryngeal disease. Few children between the ages of 2 and 13 develop hoarse voices without some underlying physical cause. It is rare for them to become hoarse or to lose their voices completely for purely functional reasons. If your own child has persistent hoarseness, take him or her to a doctor or otolaryngologist.

Other voice symptoms that may require the help of other specialists include pain associated with heavy voice use, complete loss of voice, inability to speak louder, or continued nasality. Pain while speaking, particularly after long, continued speaking, is not normal and should be investigated medically. A complete loss of voice from some physical cause might be best treated by an otolaryngologist. Loss of voice that persists without physical cause might be best treated by the speech pathologist, perhaps in collaboration with a psychologist or psychiatrist. Lack of voice loudness can usually be improved by many of the specialists who work with people with voice disorders. A nasal voice might first be evaluated by the speech pathologist who could then decide what other specialists might be needed.

In short, not all adult voice problems can be helped by reading and practicing with a book like this, although it can be a helpful supplement when you are working with other materials or treatments prescribed by one of the specialists listed below. If you need more help than we have been able to give you, if your voice problem is still there despite your efforts with our brief exercises, you need to consult an expert in the particular problem area of voice that concerns you. For your convenience we first list the specialists who treat voice disorders in alphabetical order with a brief description of what each does and then follow with a more thorough description.

Allergist	Helps control symptoms of allergy that affect voice
Audiologist	Helps when voice problems are related to hearing loss
Choir director	Helps develop better breath control for voice
Drama teacher	Helps with voice improvement and voice control
Endocrinologist	Can help with glandular and hormonal influences on voice
Inhalation therapist	Helpful if you have a breathing problem
Otolaryngologist	Treats diseases of the ear, nose, and throat
Pharmacist	Can advise on side-effects of medications on voice
Physiatrist	Prescribes exercises for breath and posture improvement
Plastic surgeon	Can treat voice resonance by surgical change of structure
Prosthodontist	Can treat nasality with dental appliances
Psychiatrist	Can help voice problems caused by anxiety and stage fright
Psychologist	Can help voice problems related to poor self-image

Speech pathologist	Provides voice evaluation and therapy for voice problems
Speech therapist	Another name for speech pathologist
Voice coach	Can improve the singing and/or speaking voice
Voice pathologist	Another name for speech pathologist
Voice scientist	An expert in the mechanisms of normal voice

Now let us look more thoroughly at each of the specialists with whom we might consult.

Allergist

An allergist is a medical doctor with a board certified specialty in allergy who diagnoses and treats various allergies. Many ear-nose-throat doctors (see Otolaryngologist) also have a special interest in allergies related to voice. For problems of phonation and resonance that only seem present during the time of an allergy, the allergist often can be most helpful in reducing these voice symptoms.

Audiologist

The audiologist is in the same profession as the speech pathologist and should be certified as a clinical audiologist by the American Speech-Language-Hearing Association (ASHA). The audiologist tests hearing and provides habilitative services, such as fitting hearing aids for people with hearing problems. Some problems of hoarseness and faulty resonance can be the direct result of hearing loss. Anyone who suspects that he or she may have a hearing loss should consult an audiologist or an otolaryngologist.

Choir Director

A choir director may be of special help if you have problems coordinating your breathing with your speaking voice. Obviously, if you have a singing problem the choir director can be helpful. But many choir directors know more about breath control and talking than many of the other specialists listed above. Since choir directors have varied backgrounds, you might ask around in your community for the names of the better choir directors.

Drama Teacher

Sometimes the local high school or college drama teacher can be of great help for the person who wants some voice help. An experienced drama coach or teacher can help develop better breathing technique for a better voice. Drama teachers often use mental imagery, encouraging their pupils to develop particular mental states as a preparation for developing a particular voice. Some theater voice techniques can markedly improve your speaking voice for talking in front of groups.

Endocrinologist

An endocrinologist is a physician with board certification in endocrinology, the study of the internal secretions and endocrine glands of the body, such as the thyroid and pituitary glands. Occasionally voice problems are related to problems of glandular or hormonal imbalance, and these are often successfully treated by the endocrinologist.

Inhalation Therapist

The growing number of people with respiratory problems (often related to a history of excessive smoking) has resulted in the emergence of the medically related specialty of inhalation therapy. For the occasional voice patient with a breathing problem, such as emphysema, the inhalation therapist can often be of greater help than any other specialist. An inhalation therapist is usually recommended by the family physician.

Otolaryngologist

The otolaryngologist is a physician with advanced training in the diagnosis and treatment of ear, nose, and throat (ENT) diseases and disorders. The patient who has continued hoarseness for more than 10 days should consult an ENT doctor for a throat examination. Speech pathologists and audiologists work closely with otolaryngologists. If the voice problem is related to disease of the vocal mechanisms, the ENT doctor would provide the primary treatment. If faulty voice usage appears to be the primary problem, the otolaryngologist will usually refer the patient to a speech pathologist for therapy.

Pharmacist

Many people do not realize that pharmacists have more knowledge about drugs and their primary and side effects than any other specialty. If a physician prescribes a medication for a particular medical problem, that drug could also cause some shortness of breath, excessive drying of mouth, or some other symptom that can directly affect voice. Consult your local pharmacist about the medications you take. Ask if there are possible side effects that might affect the way you sound. Sometimes changing from one medication to another can have a profound effect on voice.

Physiatrist

The physiatrist is a medical doctor who has completed a residency in rehabilitative medicine. He or she often heads a hospital department that may have different names such as Physical Medicine, Rehabilitation, Adaptive Medicine, or Restorative Medicine. Some voice problems are related to accidents and falls that have perhaps injured the back, neck, or head. The physiatrist often can prescribe exercise programs that will improve breathing control and body posture, which may help produce a better voice.

Plastic Surgeon

The plastic surgeon is concerned with the repair and restoration of absent, injured, or deformed parts of the body. When someone has a nasality problem related to a deformed palate or throat, the plastic surgeon often can correct the defect so that the nasality will diminish. Usually, even after surgical correction of the palate, voice therapy with a speech pathologist is required to develop normal vocal resonance.

Prosthodontist

The prosthodontist is a dentist who specializes in the construction and fitting of dentures, retainers, and palatal lifts (a device that lifts up paralyzed palates). For the occasional person with some kind of neurological problem such as stroke or disease, the prosthodontist can create an appliance that may reduce vocal nasality. The person with a cleft palate can often profit from the same kind of appliance, which can prevent the escape of air and voice through the nose and divert it out through the mouth. For the person who has a problem with false teeth, the prosthodontist is perhaps the dental specialist best able to help.

Psychiatrist

The psychiatrist is a medical doctor with a specialty interest in mental and psychological disorders. For problems of anxiety, depression, or stage fright the psychiatrist uses behavioral techniques (interview, therapy) and medical techniques (drugs) to help patients cope with their problems.

When people feel better about themselves and feel happier, their improved mood state is usually heard in their voices. People with voice problems who have difficulty relating to other people may profit from seeing a psychiatrist.

Psychologist

Most certified and licensed psychologists have a Ph.D. degree. The psychologist tests and treats patients with psychological problems such as anxiety, nervousness, and phobias. Psychologists usually offer both group and individual therapy, using various counseling and therapy techniques. People who have voice problems related to anxiety and stress in particular situations may find the psychologist's services invaluable.

Speech Pathologist

These specialists, officially called speech-language pathologists by their certifying association, the American Speech-Language-Hearing Association (ASHA), have advanced graduate training in the diagnosis and treatment of various communication disorders. Various voice pathologies, such as hoarseness related to vocal nodules or polyps, are the kind of disorders that the speech pathologist treats. Speech pathologists also have good success in treating the individual with problems of hoarseness, nasality, poor voice loudness and quality, and voice difficulties related to stage fright.

Speech Therapist

The same professional as a speech pathologist. The term *therapist* is no longer used by ASHA.

Voice Coach

The voice coach is primarily interested in the professional user of voice, such as the actor, lecturer, or singer. The experience and training of voice coaches varies. Some are former performers themselves who now specialize in working with clients in the same area of performance. Others may have specialized training in voice, and advanced degrees, and work with anyone who feels the need for voice improvement. The voice coach is often successful in increasing the loudness and improving the quality of problem voices.

Voice Pathologist

While there is no one specialty called "voice pathologist," some otolaryngologists and some speech pathologists who specialize in voice disorders sometimes designate themselves as voice pathologists.

Voice Scientist

A voice scientist is usually a doctoral level person trained in studying the various aspects of normal voice: respiration, phonation (voicing), and resonance. Although the primary interest of voice scientists is research, some are also clinically certified as either otolaryngologists or speech pathologists.

Rather than looking for a voice specialist in the yellow pages of a telephone directory or calling someone on a random hunch, ask around in your community to find knowledgeable voice people. A local medical school or university program in speech-language pathology could direct you to the best specialist for your voice problem. Other good sources of information are your doctor or the speech pathologists in a local hospital or in the schools. If you live in a small town, you might have to travel to a larger city to see a voice specialist who knows something about your problem. In the city, be sure to consult with someone who has demonstrated experience in working with people with voice problems.

Finally, a good source of information for voice problems and their treatment are the national organizations listed below. If you send them a letter of inquiry describing your problem and the need for names of specialists in your town or city, you should promptly receive a list of names of certified, well-trained specialists.

American Academy of Otolaryngology/Head and Neck Surgery
1101 Vermont Avenue N.W., Suite 302
Washington, DC 20005

American Speech-Language-Hearing Association
10801 Rockville Pike
Rockville, MD 20852

The Voice Foundation
157 East 61st Street
New York, NY 10021

Index